Free DVD · FREE · Free DVD

Essential Test Tips Video from Trivium Test Prep

Dear Customer,

Thank you for purchasing from Trivium Test Prep! Whether you're looking to join the military, get into college, or advance your career, we're honored to be a part of your journey.

To show our appreciation (and to help you relieve a little of that test-prep stress), we're offering a **FREE** *CDCES Essential Test Tips* **Video** by Trivium Test Prep. Our video includes 35 test preparation strategies that will help keep you calm and collected before and during your big exam. All we ask is that you email us your feedback and describe your experience with our product. Amazing, awful, or just so-so: we want to hear what you have to say!

To receive your **FREE** *CDCES Essential Test Tips* **Video**, please email us at 5star@ triviumtestprep.com. Include "Free 5 Star" in the subject line and the following information in your email:

1. The title of the product you purchased.

2. Your rating from 1 – 5 (with 5 being the best).

3. Your feedback about the product, including how our materials helped you meet your goals and ways in which we can improve our products.

4. Your full name and shipping address so we can send your **FREE** *CDCES Essential Test Tips* **Video**.

If you have any questions or concerns please feel free to contact us directly at 5star@triviumtestprep.com.

Thank you, and good luck with your studies!

CDCES Exam Prep

2 Practice Tests and Study Guide for the
Certified Diabetes Care and Education Specialist
[2nd Edition]

Jeremy Downs

TABLE OF CONTENTS

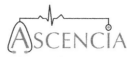

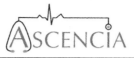

ONLINE RESOURCES

Trivium includes online resources with the purchase of this study guide to help you fully prepare for the exam.

Review Questions

Need more practice? Our review questions use a variety of formats to help you memorize key terms and concepts.

Flash Cards

Trivium's flash cards allow you to review important terms easily on your computer or smartphone.

Cheat Sheets

Review the core skills you need to master the exam with easy-to-read Cheat Sheets.

From Stress to Success

Watch "From Stress to Success," a brief but insightful YouTube video that offers the tips, tricks, and secrets experts use to score higher on the exam.

Feedback

Let us know what you think!

Access these materials at: ascenciatestprep.com/cdces-online-resources

Introduction

Congratulations on choosing to take the Certified Diabetes Care and Education Specialist (CDCES) exam! Passing this exam is an important step forward in your health care career, and we're excited to get you ready for exam day.

The CDCES Certification Process

The CDCES exam is developed by the Certification Board for Diabetes Care and Education (CBDCE) as part of its certification program for health care workers. The CDCES exam measures the knowledge necessary to provide care, education, and support to people with diabetes. Eligibility for the CDCES exam has three components:

1. **Discipline Requirements:** licensure, registration, or certification in one of the following disciplines:

   - physician
   - physician's assistant
   - registered nurse
   - pharmacist
   - podiatrist
   - clinical psychologist
   - occupational therapist
   - physical therapist
   - exercise physiologist
   - optometrist
   - dietitian or dietitian nutritionist
   - health educator
   - social worker

2. **Professional Experience:** a minimum of two years of professional practice and 1,000 hours (within a five-year period)* of providing diabetes care or education

3. **Continuing Education:** at least 15 hours of continuing education within two years before applying for certification

*There are two pathways candidates can choose when pursuing their CDCES: the standard pathway and the unique qualifications pathway. The requirements for each pathway are as follows:

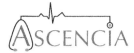

Standard Pathway

- a minimum of 200 hours of DCE experience over a one-year period
- a grand total of at least 1,000 hours of DCE experience over a five-year period

Unique Qualifications Pathway

- a minimum of 200 hours of DCE experience over a one-year period
- a grand total of at least 2,000 hours of DCE experience over a five-year period

You can apply to take the CDCES exam through the CBDCE website (https://www.cbdce.org/). Please note that you will need to submit proof of eligibility. The CBDCE website provides a handbook which contains an assessment to gauge whether you meet the prerequisites to sit for the exam. Once approved, you will receive an email with instructions for scheduling your exam. The exam must be taken within 90 days of having your application approved. It can be taken at PSI testing centers or on a personal computer using live remote online proctoring.

The CDCES Exam

When taking the CDCES exam, you will have four hours to complete 175 multiple-choice questions. Only 150 questions will be scored; the other 25 questions are pretest items included by the test makers to gauge their appropriateness for future exams. However, these pretest items will not be specified, so you must answer all questions on the exam. Since there is no penalty for incorrect answers, you should answer every question on the exam—even if you aren't sure if you are correct.

The CDCES exam content outline is broken down into three sections:

- Assessment
- Care and Education Interventions
- Standards and Practices

Within these three sections, questions are broken down as described in the following table. Visit the CBDCE website to view the full test plan.

Section and Subsections	Number of Questions
Assessment (37 total)	
Physical and Psychosocial	12
Self-Management Behaviors and Knowledge	15
Learning	10
Care and Education Interventions (105 total)	
Disease Process and Approach to Treatment	22
Individualized Education Plan	17

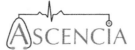

Section and Subsections	Number of Questions
Person-Centered Education on Self-Care Behaviors	58
Evaluation, Documentation, and Follow-up	8
Standards and Practices (8 total)	
includes content concerning national and practice standards, DEI, and population health strategies	8
GRAND TOTAL	**150 scored questions + 25 pretest (unscored) questions**

CDCES Exam Scoring

If you take the exam at a testing center, you will receive your score report from the proctor at the end of the exam. Candidates using live remote online proctoring will see their scores on the screen after completing the exam.

Your CDCES exam score report will contain a raw score, which is simply the number of questions you answered correctly. The raw score is converted to a scaled score, which ranges from 0 to 99. A scaled score of 70 is required to pass the exam. The number of questions you will need to answer correctly to receive a scaled score of 70 will vary with different exam formats. If you do not pass the exam, you may apply to retake the test. There is no limit on the number of times you can retake the exam.

Using This Book

This book is divided into two sections. The content review provides a concise review of key concepts in diabetes care, including pathophysiology, management, and diabetes education. Throughout these chapters, you'll also see Practice Questions that will help reinforce important concepts and skills.

The second part of the book includes practice tests with answer rationales: one test appears in the guide; the other appears as an online resource. You can use these tests to gauge your readiness for the exam and determine which content areas you may need to review more thoroughly. Follow the QR code at the end of the book to find the online practice test as well as other study resources.

Diabetes care and education specialists (hereafter referred to as *specialists*) are experienced health care professionals who collaborate with other members of a patient's care team to improve clinical outcomes for patients with diabetes by developing tools and curricula for their patients. They also share their knowledge with other health care professionals and help providers incorporate education about diabetes into their health care practices. These specialists should base their work on best practices and lead by using the latest teaching techniques.

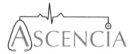

Ascencia Test Prep

With health care fields such as nursing, pharmacy, emergency care, and physical therapy becoming the fastest-growing industries in the United States, individuals looking to enter the health care industry or rise in their fields need high-quality, reliable resources. Ascencia Test Prep's study guides and test preparation materials are developed by credentialed industry professionals with years of experience in their respective fields. Ascencia recognizes that health care professionals nurture bodies and spirits, and save lives. Ascencia Test Prep's mission is to help health care workers grow.

Chapter 1 - Physical and Psychosocial Assessments

Diabetes-Relevant Health History and Social Determinants of Health

Patients with diabetes (PWD) should receive a full medical evaluation during their initial visit and again at each follow-up visit. A full evaluation includes a health history, physical examination, and laboratory testing.

General Health History

The purpose of the **health history assessment** is to collect information about the patient's general health as well as information specific to the patient's experience with diabetes symptoms and care. The diabetes care and education specialist (hereafter referred to as "specialist") should begin the interview by establishing trust with the patient. Specialists should perform the interview in a comfortable setting and discuss with patients the purpose of gathering the health history before starting the assessment.

In order to elicit full and meaningful answers from the patient, the specialist should use **open-ended questions** (i.e., those that do not have a "yes/no" answer) during the interview. For example, requesting a patient to "tell me about your pain" will yield more information than the closed question "Are you in pain?"

The components of a health history interview are discussed in Table 1.1. Note that not all of these components need to be discussed in a single interview; questions should be tailored to the patient and setting.

Helpful Hint:

The data gathered during a medical evaluation can be classified as subjective or objective. **Subjective data** are not measurable or observable and typically consist of the patient's own description of the symptoms experienced (e.g., dizziness, nausea). **Objective data** are both observable and measurable (e.g., vital signs, blood glucose levels).

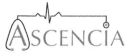

Area of Importance	Information Collected
	Table 1.1. Information Gathered in a Health History Interview (Organized by Area of Importance)
Diabetes history	• type of diabetes • duration, age, and characteristics of onset • whether the patient has ever experienced a low blood sugar reaction and how it was treated • frequency of occurrence of low blood sugar reaction • whether the patient carries a source of sugar • whether the patient has ever had to be given glucagon • whether the patient has ever experienced high blood sugar • how the patient felt and self-treated • the patient's normal daily blood sugar • whether the patient has ever been hospitalized because of diabetes
Family history	• list of family members with diabetes and history of the onset of their diabetes
Complications and comorbidities	• awareness of any diabetes complications • description of any eye, heart, kidney, dental, and/or sexual problems • indications of numbness and/or pain • any other medical conditions, such as hypertension
Surgical History	• history of surgeries the patient has undergone, including metabolic or other weight-loss surgery (e.g., bariatric)
Allergy History	• description of all known allergies, with a particular emphasis on insulin-related allergies
Behavioral factors	• description of coping mechanisms concerning caring for diabetes • description of any anxiety, helplessness, burnout, or depression • what the patient considers to be the hardest part about having diabetes • tobacco, alcohol, or drug use • physical activity and sleep patterns • eating patterns and comfort with carbohydrate counting
Medications and vaccinations	• list of current and prior medications and how the patient keeps track of these

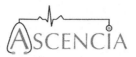

Area of Importance	Information Collected
Table 1.1. Information Gathered in a Health History Interview (Organized by Area of Importance)	
	• whether the patient takes any supplements, alternative, or OTC medications • whether the patient uses any diabetes pills or insulin, the names and dosages of these, and the frequency of use • where the patient stores insulin • whether the patient reuses syringes, and if so, how many times they are used before they are disposed • whether the patient has had the flu or pneumonia vaccination • any known complications or side effects from medications
Symptoms	• whether the patient has experienced excessive thirst, urination, or hunger; blurry vision; pain, numbness, or tingling in hands or feet; and/or unexplained weight fluctuation
Technology use	• whether the patient self-administers blood sugar tests and, if so, when and how often • patient's use of a blood glucose monitor or continuous glucose monitor • patient's use of an insulin injector or pump and review of settings on these devices
Social factors	• the patient's support system • any financial burdens that could impact care • food and housing security, access to transportation, safety at home and living situation • access to health care

Practice Questions

1. What is an open-ended question?

2. What factors should be addressed in the social factors section of the assessment interview?

Diabetes-Specific Physical Assessment and Laboratory Tests

A **physical assessment** includes checking vital signs (e.g., height, weight, blood pressure) and performing a close examination of the skin and feet to assess for diabetic complications. The provider should also palpate the thyroid to check for changes in size or firmness.

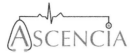

The medical evaluation should also include the following **laboratory tests**, described in further detail in Table 1.2:

- A1C (to assess glycemic control)
- kidney panel (to assess for diabetic nephropathy)
- liver panel (to assess liver function)
- thyroid function test (to assess the thyroid in patients with type 1 diabetes)
- urinalysis (to evaluate for ketones and albumin)
- lipid panel

Table 1.2. Laboratory Testing for Patients with Diabetes

Test	Description	Normal Range
Kidney Function Tests		
Blood urea nitrogen (BUN)	by-product of ammonia metabolism; filtered by the kidneys; high levels can indicate insufficient kidney function	7 – 20 mg/dL
Creatinine	product of muscle metabolism; filtered by the kidneys; high levels can indicate insufficient kidney function	0.6 – 1.2 mg/dL
BUN-to-creatinine ratio	increased ratio indicates dehydration, acute kidney injury, or gastrointestinal bleeding; decreased ratio indicates kidney damage	10:1 – 20:1
Glomerular filtration rate (GFR)	volume of fluid filtered by the renal glomerular capillaries per unit of time; decreased GFR indicates decreased kidney function	men: 100 – 130 mL/min/1.73 m^2 women: 90 – 120 mL/min/1.73 m^2 GFR <60 mL/min/1.73 m^2 is common in adults >70
Liver Function Tests		
Albumin	a protein made in the liver; low levels may indicate liver damage	3.5 – 5.0 g/dL

Chapter 1 - Physical and Psychosocial Assessments

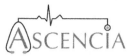

Table 1.2. Laboratory Testing for Patients with Diabetes

Test	Description	Normal Range
Alkaline phosphatase (ALP)	an enzyme found in the liver and bones; increased levels indicate liver damage	45 – 147 U/L
Alanine transaminase (ALT)	an enzyme in the liver that helps metabolize protein; increased levels indicate liver damage	7 – 55 U/L
Aspartate transaminase (AST)	an enzyme in the liver that helps metabolize proteins; increased levels indicate liver or muscle damage	8 – 48 U/L
Total protein	could indicate liver damage if low levels of total protein found	6.3 – 7.9 g/dL
Total bilirubin	produced during the breakdown of heme (haem); increased levels indicate liver damage or anemia	0.1 – 1.2 mg/dL
Thyroid Function Tests		
Thyroid stimulating hormone (TSH)	produced by the anterior pituitary gland; high TSH indicates hypothyroidism (associated with Hashimoto's thyroiditis, pituitary gland disease); low TSH indicates hyperthyroidism (associated with Graves' disease, toxic thyroid nodule)	0.5 – 5.0 mU/L
T4	produced by the thyroid gland; high levels indicate hyperthyroidism; low levels indicate hypothyroidism	0.7 – 1.9 ng/dL if taking medications that change thyroid hormone metabolism or history of thyroid cancer or pituitary disease 5.0 – 12.0 µg/dL

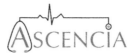

Table 1.2. Laboratory Testing for Patients with Diabetes		
Test	**Description**	**Normal Range**
T3	produced by the thyroid gland; high levels indicate hyperthyroidism; low levels indicate hypothyroidism	80 – 220 ng/dL
Urinalysis		
Ketones	indicate high blood glucose and ketoacidosis	<0.5 mmol/L
Microalbumin/creatine ratio	compares the amounts of albumin to creatinine in urine	<30

Practice Questions

3. What is the normal level of TSH?

4. What glomerular filtration rate indicates decreased kidney function for women?

Mental Health Well-Being

Managing diabetes requires complex lifestyle changes and constant monitoring that can create high levels of stress. People with diabetes (PWD) may also face pressure from family, friends, and medical practitioners that creates additional stress. Developing healthy ways to cope with this stress is an essential element of living a successful and sustainable life with diabetes.

Healthy coping is defined as a positive attitude toward diabetes and diabetes self-management. Patients who are coping well with diabetes are proactive about managing their care. They engage in behaviors that improve their quality of life and maintain healthy support networks. When patients cope with diabetes in a healthy way, they are taking a full biopsychosocial approach to their care. The elements that comprise healthy coping are listed in Table 1.3.

Table 1.3. Elements of Healthy Coping		
Biological	**Psychological**	**Social**
• medication • monitoring • dietary pattern • exercise	• generating ideas for improved care • positive self-talk • reflecting on progress	• building support networks • finding friends with diabetes or support groups

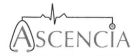

ASCENCIA

Table 1.3. Elements of Healthy Coping		
Biological	**Psychological**	**Social**
		• nurturing relationships with loved ones

Healthy coping is encouraged by building a sense of self-sufficiency in the patient. **Problem-solving skills** are key components in the development of self-sufficiency. Patients should be taught to break down problem-solving into a step-by-step process:

1. **Identify the problem.** Helping patients explore barriers to more effective diabetes care is the first step to improving their care.

2. **Understand the problem.** Once the problem is identified, patients must be able to fully define it. The better patients understand the problem, the easier it will be for them to find solutions.

3. **Generate solutions.** There are many possible solutions to problems that can arise when managing diabetes. Patients should learn how to research solutions and organize the information they find.

4. **Monitor progress.** Patients should monitor their progress as they develop and implement solutions.

5. **Evaluate solutions.** Specialists should follow up with patients to help them evaluate the success of specific solutions. Patients should also be encouraged to analyze which specific elements of a solution helped make it a success—or a challenge—to implement.

> **Helpful Hint**
>
> Healthy coping is the first ADCES7 self-care behavior and forms the foundation for diabetes self-management. Patients with poor coping strategies will likely struggle with the other self-care behaviors.

> **Helpful Hint**
>
> Healthy coping is the first ADCES7 self-care behavior and forms the foundation for diabetes self-management. Patients with poor coping strategies will likely struggle with the other self-care behaviors.

The specific techniques that will help improve coping skills in patients will depend on the problems they are facing and their specific circumstances. The management of specific elements of healthy coping are discussed in detail in the sections which follow.

Practice Questions

5. What is the definition of healthy coping in patients with diabetes?

6. What are the steps to problem-solving that patients with diabetes should learn?

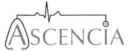

Considerations Related to Diabetes Self-Care Practices

Cognitive Dysfunction

Cognitive dysfunction is a broad term that refers to many types of cognitive functioning issues. Some common types of cognitive dysfunction include difficulties with the following:

- attention and memory (also known as brain fog)
- executive functioning (ability to do everyday tasks that require planning and sequencing)
- taking in information (learning)

Patients with diabetes (PWD) are at risk of developing cognitive dysfunction linked to poor glycemic control. The microvascular damage caused by chronic hyperglycemia affects the brain much like it does other organs, potentially altering the person's cognitive functioning. For some patients, this cycle can intensify as cognitive dysfunction makes it more difficult to manage blood glucose (BG) levels.

Patients with type 1 diabetes are also at risk for cognitive dysfunction caused by severe **hypoglycemia**, an irregular drop in blood sugar levels (blood glucose below 70 milligrams per deciliter (mg/dl). Patients with diabetes who are diagnosed at a very young age are particularly susceptible and have much higher rates of cognitive dysfunction. This dysfunction is likely caused by the great variability of BG levels during a time of rapid brain growth and development.

The American Diabetes Association (ADA) recommends the **Montreal Cognitive Assessment (MoCA)** for assessing cognitive function in PWD. The MoCA is a 30-question test that takes about 10 minutes to complete. It assesses orientation to time and place, short-term memory, executive functioning, language skills, and the ability to understand abstract ideas. This assessment is recommended because it is easy to administer and tests a wide variety of types of memory and attention.

> **Helpful Hint**:
>
> The most common types of cognitive dysfunction seen in patients with type 2 diabetes are difficulties with learning and memory.

For patients with comorbid cognitive dysfunction and diabetes, care is best focused on methods that simplify care management. The simplest way to achieve this is to minimize the number and types of treatment needed throughout the day. For example, patients who struggle to take insulin at every meal can switch to a once-daily basal insulin. Memory aids, such as pillboxes and calendar alerts, can also help patients adhere to treatment regimens.

Practice Questions

7. What tool does the ADA recommend for assessing cognitive function in patients with diabetes?

8. What type of patient is MOST at risk for cognitive dysfunction related to type 1 diabetes?

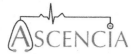

Depression

Fear, worry, and a feeling of being overwhelmed are common responses to a diabetes diagnosis; however, when those symptoms become severe, they can inhibit daily functioning. At this point, patients require further help, and a mental health diagnosis may be needed. Both depression and anxiety are common mental health issues seen in PWD.

Depression is a mood disorder characterized by depressed mood and lack of interest in previously pleasurable activities. Patients with depression may report issues with concentration, sleep, and appetite; they may also report suicidal ideation. Depression can also interfere with patients' abilities to care for themselves and manage their diabetes.

> **Helpful Hint**:
>
> Diabetes is a significant risk factor for depression. Possible reasons for this link include the emotional burden of managing diabetes, the effects of unstable blood glucose levels on the brain, and lifestyle factors that contribute to both depression and worsening diabetes (e.g., poor diet, lack of exercise).

There are two main types of depression:

- **Persistent depressive disorder** is a milder, long-term form of depression.

- **Major depressive disorder** is a more acute form of depression that can severely inhibit day-to-day functioning.

Depression is a very serious condition, but it is treatable. PWD should be regularly screened for symptoms of depression using a questionnaire such as the **Patient Health Questionnaire-9 (PHQ-9)**. If questionnaires or interviews suggest that patients have symptoms of depression, they should be referred to mental health care. They may need therapy, psychiatric intervention in the form of antidepressants, or a combination of the two to treat their depression.

Anxiety

Anxiety is the presence of excessive worry. It can be about particular things, such as a fear of hypoglycemia, or it can be a broader, nonspecific worry. Common symptoms of anxiety include irritability, memory and concentration problems, and physiological symptoms such as weakness or dizziness.

Patients who report symptoms of anxiety should be referred for mental health care. Effective anxiety treatment typically involves therapy with a licensed counselor, therapist, or psychologist to learn coping skills to manage worry and fear. It may also incorporate the use of antianxiety medications prescribed by a psychiatrist to regulate mood.

Symptoms of both depression and anxiety can be similar to symptoms caused by poor blood glucose (BG) management. Persistent hyperglycemia can affect energy levels, appetite, and sleep in ways that mimic depression. Similarly, hypoglycemia can cause many of the same symptoms seen in people with anxiety. For this reason, patients with apparent mental health issues should be closely assessed for glycemic control in addition to receiving mental health referrals.

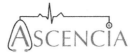

Practice Questions

9. What are some of the symptoms of depression?

10. What is the recommended treatment for a patient experiencing anxiety?

11. A diabetes care and education specialist has a patient who scores very high on the PHQ-9. What should the specialist do to help this patient?

Roles and Responsibilities of Care

Diabetes does not just affect the person with the diagnosis; it also affects the entire family. Family dynamics can become complicated as the patient's family tries to balance their own stressors with the patient's need for support.

It is common for family members to feel a great deal of fear for their loved one with diabetes, especially when they do not understand much about the disease. The best way to allay these fears is to increase education on the topic. Family members who understand how best to manage diabetes care will likely feel empowered instead of scared and be better prepared to support the patient.

Family members sometimes have unrealistic expectations about managing diabetes. When PWD do not immediately improve or meet goals, family members may become disparaging or controlling. The families often mean well, but these behaviors can lead to negative feelings, tension, and may encourage PWD to not take responsibility for their own health.

Despite these potential difficulties, PWD can benefit from family support. Seeking help from family in a way that preserves positive dynamics can be difficult; however, teaching PWD how to do so is an important part of helping them live with and manage their diabetes effectively. The following steps can help PWD communicate productively with their families about diabetes-related issues:

> 1. **Use "I" statements.** Instead of "You get on my nerves when you control my food," use "I feel annoyed when you tell me not to eat sweets."

> 2. **Acknowledge their concerns.** Family members usually have their loved one's best interests at heart. Acknowledging this can help smooth over hurt feelings or sensitivities.

> 3. **Communicate what is needed.** The best way for PWD to get what they need from family members is to ask for it. Patients can also try suggesting an alternative behavior to replace the unwanted behavior (e.g., "Instead of telling me not to eat sweets, it would help me a lot if we could make some low-sugar desserts together.")

> 4. **Thank them.** Changing behaviors is a lot of work. Patients should make sure to thank any family members willing to talk with them and work on their behavior.

> 5. **Schedule.** Creating a set schedule of check-ins can help improve communication by increasing opportunities to discuss problems when emotions are not running high.

> 6. **Review.** Changing behaviors takes time. Everyone involved needs to feel valued and listened to. If a conversation goes badly, patients should step away and try again another day.

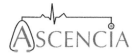

Practice Questions

12. How can specialists help decrease family members' fears for the patient?

13. What are "I" statements?

Diabetes Distress

The stress of managing diabetes can leave patients with negative feelings, such as frustration, denial, anger, and helplessness—a condition known as **diabetes distress**. This condition is different from depression in that it specifically stems from issues related to diabetes care, concerns, and support. Diabetes distress results from a combination of stressors:

- the burden of managing diabetes

- the emotional distress of having diabetes

- the fear of potentially developing complications

- low support and care

Diabetes distress can affect not only the patient but also family members and caregivers. The primary assessment tool for diabetes distress is the **diabetes distress scale**, of which there are several versions:

- **Parent-DDS**

- **Partner-DDS**

- **T1-DDS**

- **T2-DDAS**

> **Helpful Hint**
>
> Studies suggest that 30% – 40% of patients with diabetes will experience moderate to severe diabetes distress at some point during their lifetimes.

The questions on each assessment reflect the relationship to the person with diabetes (parent, partner, or self) and the type of diabetes (type 1 or type 2).

High levels of diabetes distress are associated with poor glycemic management. Individuals whose score on a diabetes distress scale is high or even moderate would benefit from speaking to a mental health professional. Care may focus on managing stress and implementing techniques to improve healthy coping, build up a stronger support network, and develop healthy habits.

Practice Questions

14. What is diabetes distress?

15. What is the best tool to assess a parent of a PWD for diabetes distress?

Cultural and Spiritual

Personal beliefs, religiosity, and spirituality can affect a person's health and treatment behaviors in a negative or positive manner. Supporting a person's spirituality in regard to diabetes management is important since it can help reduce anxiety, promote resiliency, and offer comfort. Spiritual

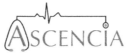

considerations can have various meanings and may include meditation, finding direction or a source of strength, or seeking a higher power through prayer. Discussions on spirituality may come naturally for others but can be uncomfortable for others. Medical professionals can use anonymous surveys to assess the comfort level of patients when discussing spirituality.

Cultural sensitivity describes an acceptance and awareness that various cultures exist. In health care, a culturally sensitive approach focuses on respecting both verbal or nonverbal interactions and communications between the patient and professional, and it encourages involved parties to express their own cultures. Cultural sensitivity relies on behavioral reinforcement, which is rooted in conditioning; reinforcement may be positive or negative. To better improve health care outcomes for culturally distinct populations, health care professionals and systems must become culturally competent.

Cultural competence is the ability of health systems to recognize a person's beliefs, diverse values, and behaviors. It is a general principle that allows one to encompass religion, ethnicity, and culture, which are all needed to optimize care for people with diabetes. Specialists must tailor treatment plans to meet the cultural, social, and linguistic needs of patients. Cultural competence focuses on behavioral change and involves a broad set of techniques. Specialists practicing cultural competence will attempt to create an understanding of how to deliver optimal care and respond to the needs of diverse populations. For example, if clinical care is not accessible to a specific community, it can indicate a lack of cultural competencies by health care workers in that community. Questions such as "Why did one community get care options but another did not?" must be asked in order to approach health care treatment options with cultural competence. In order to reduce health inequities, health professionals must make effective and evidence-based care accessible to diverse populations.

Practice Question

16. How does cultural competence differ from cultural sensitivity?

Language

Many professional groups, medical journals, and diabetes organizations have advocated for improved language concerning diabetes. Language has the power of persuasion and the ability to reinforce/change a person's beliefs and stereotypes, which can be positive or negative. Specialists should focus on inclusive language that emphasizes what a person can do and provides motivation and support for the person with diabetes. Language must be neutral and nonjudgmental, free from stigma, and factual. According to researchers in diabetes psychology, patients with diabetes will experience greater emotional distress compared to those without diabetes. One source of distress is the type of language that refers to diabetes: how written and verbal language is used will reflect and shape a person's thoughts, behaviors, and beliefs. Based on a publication in *The New England Journal of Medicine*, researchers have suggested the use of verbal statements that support quality of life. For example, instead of saying, "What is the matter with you?" the phrase can be substituted with "What matters to you?"

Another language consideration utilized by professional groups is to create a flourishing mindset for patients that builds on their positive experiences and focuses on their health. Using open dialogues, specialists can identify and celebrate the successful behaviors that patients display in everyday life as opposed to centering on illness-related and correctional behaviors.

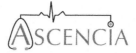

The UK National Health Service published a document called "Language matters: Language and Diabetes," which recognizes how health care professionals can use language to significantly impact health outcomes for patients with diabetes. The document sets forth basic principles for good practice regarding interactions between health care professionals and patients with diabetes. For example, specialists should strive to be trust-builders who are empathetic, empowering, person-centered, culturally competent, encouraging, clear, and reassuring. Specialists—and all health care professionals—must aim to convey information in ways that are less stigmatizing, demanding, authoritarian, and judgmental.

Clinicians must also assess and measure the cognitive function of patients who may have cognitive impairments. Patients with cognitive or language impairments may have difficulty expressing themselves verbally and/or comprehending speech. Consequently, clinicians must implement strategies that are optimized towards the self-care of the patient.

Practice Question

17. To what document can a specialist refer when determining the best language to use when interacting with both colleagues and PWD?

Fears and Myths

Many patients will experience fear and anxiety as they learn to manage their diabetes. Patients will also encounter common myths about diabetes that can make care more challenging. Specialists should work with patients to alleviate these fears and correct misinformation that impedes diabetes care:

- **Fear of hypoglycemia or hyperglycemia:** PWD may have a fear of acute hypo- or hyperglycemia, both of which can put the patient at risk of health complications, and, in extreme cases, loss of consciousness or even death. The best way to help patients with these fears is through education and preparation. Some helpful practices for the patient include

    o tracking BG—particularly through variations in dietary patterns and activity—to better understand how hypo- or hyperglycemic episodes can occur;
    o being prepared with snacks, glucose, and extra insulin;
    o educating family and friends about how to help in the event of a hypo- or hyperglycemic episode; and
    o wearing a medical bracelet that can alert health care providers to the patient's condition in the case of an emergency.

- **Fear of needles:** A fear of needles may predate a diabetes diagnosis, or it may develop as patients face constant needle usage. Fears and intense phobias are best managed through gradual exposure, although this can be difficult when the need for needle usage is constant. Some other ways to help patients cope with a fear of needles can include

    o using a continuous glucose monitor or insulin pump;
    o asking a family member or friend to administer insulin;
    o practicing inserting needles into oranges, which creates a sensation similar to piercing skin; and
    o asking family or friends to be around to hold a hand or offer words of encouragement.

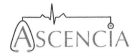

- **Fear of gaining weight:** Insulin allows cells to process and store glucose, which can lead to weight gain. Patients who are beginning an insulin regimen may worry about this weight gain; they may be concerned about the health outcomes associated with being overweight, or they may be facing significant social pressure to lose weight.

  - Patients should be reassured that some weight gain is normal and signals that the treatment is working.
  - Specialists can work with these patients to adjust their dietary patterns, activity, and antidiabetic agent regimens to balance possible weight gain.

- **Myths about the cause of diabetes:** There are many myths about the causes of diabetes. Often these myths place the blame for a diabetes diagnosis on the patient. For example, people may believe that diabetes is caused by eating sugar, being overweight, or not exercising enough. Because lifestyle factors can increase the risk of type 2 diabetes and gestational diabetes mellitus, patients with these conditions in particular may feel that they did something to cause the disease. Specialists should explain to patients that a diabetes diagnosis is not their "fault" and provide education on lifestyle changes without placing blame on the patient.

> **Helpful Hint**:
>
> Surveys have found that one in three women with type 1 diabetes have restricted insulin to lose weight.

Practice Questions

18. What is the BEST way to help a patient overcome a fear of needles?

19. How can the diabetes care and education specialist help a patient who has a fear of acute hypoglycemia?

Chapter 1 Answer Key

1. An open-ended question is a question that does not have a yes/no answer.

2. The social factors part of the interview should address the patient's support system, their financial situation, transportation access, food and housing security, and their safety at home.

3. The normal level of TSH is 0.5 to 5.0 mU/L.

4. A GFR below 90 mL/min/1.73 m2 indicates decreased renal function in women.

5. Healthy coping is the development of a positive attitude toward diabetes and diabetes

self-management.

6. The steps to problem-solving are (1) identify the problem, (2) understand the problem, (3) generate solutions, (4) monitor progress, and (5) evaluate solutions.

7. The ADA recommends the Montreal Cognitive Assessment (MoCA) to assess cognitive

functioning in patients with diabetes.

8. Very young patients with type 1 diabetes have a higher risk of developing cognitive dysfunction.

9. Symptoms of depression include depressed mood and lack of interest in previously pleasurable activities; issues with concentration, sleep, and appetite; and suicidal ideation.

10. To treat anxiety, mental health experts recommend counseling and antianxiety medication.

11. The patient should be referred to mental health services for diagnosis and treatment.

12. Fear often stems from a lack of knowledge or understanding about a topic; increased education can lessen fear about diabetes care management.

13. "I" statements are statements in which the focus is on the feelings of the speaker instead of the actions of the listener.

14. Diabetes distress refers to negative feelings that arise from the stress of managing diabetes.

15. Diabetes distress is assessed through the use of the diabetes distress scale (DDS). The most appropriate version for a parent would be the Parent-DDS.

16. Cultural competence is the ability of health systems to recognize a person's beliefs, diverse values, and behaviors whereas cultural sensitivity describes an acceptance and awareness that various cultures exist.

17. Specialists should refer to *Language matters: Language and Diabetes*, which is a document published by the UK National Health Service; it sets forth basic principles for good practice regarding interactions between health care professionals and patients with diabetes.

18. Repeated exposure is the best way to help a patient overcome phobias, including a fear of needles.

19. Education and preparation are the best ways to alleviate patient fears about hypoglycemia. Patients can be encouraged to track blood glucose (BG) levels, be prepared with glucose, educate friends and family, and wear a medical bracelet.

Chapter 2 - Self-Management Knowledge

Disease Process and Pathophysiology

Diabetes is *characterized* by deficiencies in carbohydrate metabolism that result in **hyperglycemia** (high blood glucose levels). Hyperglycemia may be caused by a lack of insulin secretion, action, or both.

Diabetes is *categorized* based on the underlying etiology of the hyperglycemia. Here is a summary of the different types of diabetes:

1. **Type 1 diabetes**
   - Description: An autoimmune disease in which the immune system destroys beta cells in the pancreas, resulting in a lack of insulin production.
   - Populations at Highest Risk: Children ages 4 – 6 and 10 – 14 with a family history of diabetes.
   - Approximate Percentage of Diagnosed Cases in the US: 6%

2. **Type 2 diabetes**
   - Description: Progressive loss of beta cell function, often occurring alongside insulin resistance.
   - Populations at Highest Risk: People aged >45 years who are obese with genetic predisposition or lifestyle risk factors (e.g., poor dietary pattern, lack of activity).
   - Approximate Percentage of Diagnosed Cases in the US: 90%

3. **Gestational diabetes**
   - Description: Inability of beta cells to compensate for increased insulin resistance caused by pregnancy.
   - Populations at Highest Risk: Pregnant women in the second or third trimester who are obese and have genetic or lifestyle risk factors similar to those for type 2 diabetes.
   - Approximate Percentage of Diagnosed Cases in the US: N/A

4. **Monogenic diabetes**
   - Description: Group of conditions caused by genetic defects that impair beta cell functioning.
   - Populations at Highest Risk: People with a family history of monogenic diabetes.
   - Approximate Percentage of Diagnosed Cases in the US: 4%

5. **Pancreatic diabetes (type 3c)**
   - Description: Damage to the exocrine pancreas.

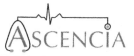

- Populations at Highest Risk: People with disease of the pancreas or who have had pancreatic tissue removed.

6. **Drug-induced diabetes**

- Description: Use of drugs that affect insulin secretion or action.

- Populations at Highest Risk: Use of high-risk drugs, including corticosteroids, antipsychotics, and immunological drugs.

Practice Questions

1. How is diabetes characterized?

2. How is diabetes categorized?

Honeymoon Period and Dawn Phenomenon

After diagnosis, patients with type 1 diabetes may experience a "honeymoon" stage. Known as the **honeymoon period**, this stage describes when the pancreatic beta cells create a small amount of insulin. As time passes and the honeymoon stage wanes, the pancreas produces less insulin, and individuals with type 1 diabetes will have an increasing need for exogenous insulin. Consequently, the management needs of type 1 diabetes will increase, and patients will have the continual expectation of managing their diabetes as they undergo developmental, physical, emotional, and behavioral changes.

Children in the **honeymoon period** of T1D may require little or no insulin. During this brief period of remission, the pancreas produces enough endogenous insulin to keep blood glucose near normal levels. This period usually lasts between 6 months and 2 years; when it ends, these patients will require higher levels of exogenous insulin. Parents of pediatric patients with diabetes must work with the specialist to help monitor the pediatric patient's changes related to puberty in order to ensure that glycemic levels do not worsen. Furthermore, it is recommended that there be constant consultation with young patients, their parents, and diabetes management teams in regard to stress management, nutrition, exercise, and insulin adjustment. Without consultation, the development of acute complications, hyperglycemia, and glucose fluctuations can occur.

High BG early in the morning is common for PWD. This early morning spike will often subside with few impacts on the patient; however, frequent high morning glucose can increase A1C. There are three main causes of early morning hyperglycemia:

- Food and antidiabetic agents can lead to early morning hyperglycemia. Patients whose basal/long-acting insulin levels are too low may experience hyperglycemia. Bedtime meals and snacks may also lead to overnight hyperglycemia that persists until morning.

- **Dawn phenomenon** (discussed below) occurs as a result of hormones released during the waking process, including cortisol and growth hormone. These hormones increase blood glucose levels, typically between 2:00 and 8:00 a.m.

> **Helpful Hint:**
> Studies using continuous glucose monitoring have shown that the Somogyi effect is quite rare. Most cases of early morning hyperglycemia are the result of the dawn phenomenon or are related to food or antidiabetic agents.

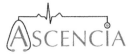

- The **Somogyi effect** is when a drop in blood glucose in the evening causes a rebound effect, resulting in hyperglycemia in the early morning.

Diabetes researchers observed dawn phenomena for individuals who undergo early morning fasting (between 4 a.m. to 8 a.m.). **Dawn phenomena** describes when, during these early morning hours, growth hormones and cortisol signal the liver to produce glucose, leading to unexpectedly high blood glucose levels. The phenomena are attributed to reduced peripheral and hepatic insulin sensitivity and nocturnal spikes of growth hormone. Consequently, patients with diabetes will wake up with symptoms such as increased hunger, thirst, or urination, in addition to the possibility of having headaches and blurred vision. Some studies have indicated that using basal insulin via continuous subcutaneous insulin infusion (CSII), known as insulin therapy, combined with continuous glucose monitoring (CGM) can be effective for dawn phenomena management.

Practice Question

3. What physiological processes cause early morning hyperglycemia in patients with dawn phenomenon?

Type 1 Diabetes

Type 1 diabetes is an autoimmune disease that results in the destruction of pancreatic beta cells. The resulting lack of insulin production leads to persistent hyperglycemia. Without medical care, type 1 diabetes leads to **diabetic ketoacidosis (DKA)**, a life-threatening condition characterized by severe hyperglycemia and ketoacidosis.

Symptoms of type 1 diabetes typically appear in children ages 4 to 6 and 10 to 14 (early puberty). Patients with undiagnosed type 1 diabetes present with hyperglycemia; around 50 percent of children with undiagnosed type 1 diabetes present with DKA. Common symptoms include "the three Ps of diabetes":

- polyuria
- polydipsia
- polyphagia

Polyuria (excessive urination) is the result of osmotic diuresis. Excess glucose in the blood cannot be reabsorbed by the kidneys. The resulting osmotic gradient pulls excess fluid into the renal tubules, resulting in high volumes of urine. Excess urination causes dehydration and **polydipsia** (excessive thirst).

Polyphagia (excessive hunger) occurs when the lack of insulin prevents uptake of glucose into cells, leaving cells starved for energy. The inability of cells to use glucose can lead to weight loss, fatigue, and weakness. The body may also begin to break down fat and muscle.

Helpful Hint:
While type 1 diabetes most commonly develops in childhood, it can also occur in adults.

Type 1 diabetes is characterized by the presence of **pancreatic autoantibodies**, markers that appear when pancreatic beta cells are damaged. Autoantibodies are present in type 1 diabetes and absent in forms of diabetes resulting from non-autoimmune causes. While patients with suspected diabetes are not routinely tested for pancreatic autoantibodies, testing may be

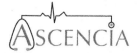

ordered to confirm a diagnosis of type 1 diabetes or to screen high-risk patients. Type 1 diabetes develops in three stages:

- **Stage 1:** Autoantibodies are present but patients are euglycemic and asymptomatic.

- **Stage 2:** Patients are hyperglycemic but still asymptomatic.

- **Stage 3:** Patients are hyperglycemic and present with symptoms (the three Ps).

Diagnosis of type 1 diabetes is based on a plasma glucose (PG) or A1C test:

- In patients with symptoms of hyperglycemia, a random plasma glucose ≥200 mg/dL is sufficient for diagnosis.

- In asymptomatic individuals, diabetes is diagnosed at

    - A1C ≥6.5%,
    - fasting plasma glucose (FPG) ≥126 mg/dL, or
    - 2-hr PG ≥200 mg/dL.

In the US, type 1 diabetes is most common among non-Hispanic White people. Men and women are affected equally. Risk factors for type 1 diabetes include

- family history (i.e., genetic predisposition);

- the presence of pancreatic autoantibodies; and

- viral exposure, including fetal exposure to Coxsackievirus or enterovirus during pregnancy

Helpful Hint:

If hyperglycemia develops rapidly, an A1C may show normal results. In this situation, plasma glucose should be used to confirm diagnosis.

Practice Questions

4. What are the THREE most common presenting symptoms of hyperglycemia?

5. What is the level of fasting plasma glucose necessary to diagnose diabetes?

6. What A1C level indicates diabetes?

7. A patient with pancreatic autoantibodies and asymptomatic hyperglycemia is in which stage of type 1 diabetes?

8. In a patient presenting with classic symptoms of diabetes, what random plasma glucose level is sufficient to diagnose diabetes?

Type 2 Diabetes

Type 2 diabetes is a progressive disease caused by increasing dysfunction of pancreatic beta cells, often accompanied by insulin resistance. The pathophysiology of type 2 diabetes is complex and not fully understood. Decreased insulin secretion by beta cells is progressive and related to many factors, including genetic predisposition and cell exposure to chronic inflammation and high glucose levels.

Insulin resistance occurs when the body does not respond normally to insulin, preventing glucose from entering cells. It is highly correlated to obesity and is exacerbated by poor dietary patterns and aging.

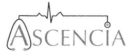

Diagnosis of type 2 diabetes uses the same criteria as type 1 diabetes: patients with hyperglycemia caused by type 2 diabetes will also present with polyuria, polydipsia, and polyphagia; however, patients may not recognize these symptoms since they can develop gradually over many years.

People who are developing type 2 diabetes may pass through a phase called **prediabetes**. This condition is characterized by blood glucose levels that are high but do not meet the threshold for diagnosis of diabetes. Screening for prediabetes is done through a blood glucose test.

> **Helpful Hint**:
>
> Insulin resistance alone does not cause type 2 diabetes, but it can worsen the progressive dysfunction of beta cells.

Table 2.2. Diagnosis of Prediabetes and Type 2 Diabetes

Test	Prediabetes	Type 2 Diabetes
FPG	100 – 125 mg/dL	≥126 mg/dL
2-hr PG	140 – 199 mg/dL	≥200 mg/dL
A1C	5.7% – 6.4%	≥6.5%
Random plasma glucose	not used for prediabetic screening	≥200 mg/dL (for symptomatic patients)

Prediabetes does not require medical management but is a significant risk factor for developing type 2 diabetes. Changes in dietary patterns and activity levels can reduce the risk of progression to type 2 diabetes in people with prediabetes. According to American Diabetes Association (ADA) guidelines, the following people should be screened for prediabetes:

- adults with a body mass index (BMI) of ≥25 kg/m2 and one other significant risk factor for cardiovascular disease (e.g., family history, cardiovascular disease, hypertension, or hyperlipidemia)

- people with a history of gestational diabetes (every three years)

- people with a history of prediabetes (yearly)

- people aged 35 years and older (minimum of every three years)

The most significant risk factor for type 2 diabetes is obesity, particularly when fat is primarily distributed in the abdominal area. Other risk factors include a sedentary lifestyle (i.e., sitting for more than 90 minutes at a time or little to no moderate to vigorous activity in the past 30 days); a high-calorie dietary pattern; and a history of gestational diabetes, hypertension, or hyperlipidemia. Genetic predisposition and family history also play significant roles in the risk of developing type 2 diabetes.

Pacific Islanders, Alaska Natives, and Native Americans are the ethnic groups with the highest rates of type 2 diabetes. The ethnic group with the lowest rate of type 2 diabetes is non-Hispanic Whites. Type 2 diabetes is more common in individuals over age forty-five, and men are at a higher risk than women.

> **Did You Know**?
>
> Thirty-nine percent of people with type 2 diabetes have at least one parent who also has type 2 diabetes.

Chapter 2 - Self-Management Knowledge

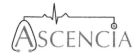

Practice Questions

9. What range of A1C indicates prediabetes?

10. What type of fat distribution is correlated with a higher risk for type 2 diabetes?

11. Why are patients with undiagnosed type 2 diabetes less likely to report symptoms of polyuria, polydipsia, and polyphagia?

12. How often should a 38-year-old with no risk factors for diabetes be screened for prediabetes?

13. Which two physiological processes cause type 2 diabetes?

Gestational Diabetes

Gestational diabetes mellitus (GDM) is characterized by hyperglycemia that develops during the second or third trimester of pregnancy. The physiological processes that underlie GDM are similar to those that lead to type 2 diabetes. Insulin resistance increases during pregnancy as a result of placental hormones and metabolic changes. When beta cells cannot secrete enough insulin to compensate for the insulin resistance, the pregnant person's glucose levels rise.

Helpful Hint:

Elevated blood glucose in the first trimester of pregnancy is indicative of preexisting type 1 or 2 diabetes, not GDM.

Hyperglycemia during pregnancy is linked to increased risk for preeclampsia, fetal abnormalities, and preterm delivery. Babies born to mothers with GDM are also typically larger, increasing the likelihood of cesarean section and related morbidities. Medical management to maintain euglycemia during pregnancy reduces the risk for these outcomes.

Gestational diabetes is usually asymptomatic, so both the ADA and the American College of Obstetricians and Gynecologists (ACOG) recommend that all pregnant patients be screened for GDM. Screening can occur as a one- or two-step process, as described in Table 2.3.

Table 2.3. Diagnosis of Gestational Diabetes

One-Step Process	Two-Step Process
	Step 1
	50 g glucose loading test (GLT) at 24 – 28 weeks
75 g oral glucose tolerance test (OGTT) at 24 – 28 weeks; GDM is diagnosed for the following findings:	If 1-hour plasma glucose ≥130 mg/dL, administer step 2.
	Step 2
• fasting ≥92 mg/dL • 1 hour ≥180 mg/dL • 2 hour ≥153 mg/dL	100 g OGTT GDM is diagnosed for the following findings: • fasting ≥95 mg/dL • 1 hour ≥180 mg/dL • 2 hour ≥155 mg/dL

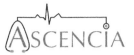

Table 2.3. Diagnosis of Gestational Diabetes	
One-Step Process	**Two-Step Process**
	• 3 hour ≥140 mg/dL Note: Threshold for diagnosis varies for different guidelines. The lowest threshold is given here.

Risk factors for GDM are similar to those for type 2 diabetes. Patients who are obese and have risk factors for cardiovascular disease (e.g., hypertension, hyperlipidemia) are at higher risk for GDM. Ethnic groups at higher risk include African Americans, Hispanics, Asians, and Native Americans.

Patients diagnosed with GDM should be screened at 4 – 12 weeks postpartum to rule out the presence of other types of diabetes. Because the underlying mechanisms are similar, people diagnosed with GDM are at high risk of developing type 2 diabetes; around 50% of people diagnosed with GDM go on to develop type 2 diabetes later in life. Patients diagnosed with GDM should be screened every three years for type 2 diabetes.

Practice Questions

14. When should pregnant patients be screened for gestational diabetes?

15. Uncontrolled hyperglycemia during pregnancy increases the risk for what conditions in the mother and baby?

16. Why is continued screening for diabetes suggested for patients diagnosed with gestational diabetes?

Other Types of Diabetes

Monogenic diabetes is a group of disorders caused by defects to specific genes that result in beta cell dysfunction. It typically presents in patients younger than twenty-five who have family histories of monogenic diabetes. Patients will be hyperglycemic, but no pancreatic autoantibodies will be present. Monogenic diabetes can be diagnosed through genetic testing. Management of monogenic diabetes is similar to management of other types of diabetes, with some variations requiring insulin and others requiring only antidiabetic agents or lifestyle changes.

Diabetes may also be caused by damage to the pancreas, a condition called **pancreatic diabetes**, **type 3c diabetes**, or **diabetes in the context of disease of the exocrine pancreas**. Common causes of pancreatic diabetes include cystic fibrosis, pancreatitis, hemochromatosis, and resection of pancreatic tissue. Pancreatic diabetes differs from other types of diabetes because alpha cells are also damaged, placing patients at risk of both hypo- and hyperglycemia.

> **Helpful Hint**:
>
> **Maturity-onset diabetes of the young (MODY)** refers to a form of monogenic diabetes caused by defects in the HNF4A gene. The different types of monogenic diabetes are sometimes referred to as MODY subtypes.

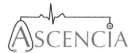
Drug-induced diabetes can be caused by a range of drugs that inhibit insulin secretion or action or that increase glucose production in the liver. This type of diabetes usually occurs in people who have genetic or other risk factors. Drugs that may induce diabetes include the following:

- corticosteroids (most common)
- antipsychotics
- statins
- HIV retrovirals
- chemotherapeutic agents
- growth hormone therapy

Practice Questions

17. How is monogenic diabetes diagnosed?

18. What are common causes of pancreatic tissue damage that can result in pancreatic diabetes?

19. Which type of drug is most commonly responsible for drug-induced diabetes?

Monitoring and Data Collection

Glucose Testing

Blood glucose levels can be measured using several different laboratory tests. A **random plasma glucose** is taken at any time. Because blood glucose levels vary with food and activity (see Figure 2.1.), this test does not provide precise information about glucose metabolism. It is usually only used to diagnosis hypo- or hyperglycemia in symptomatic patients.

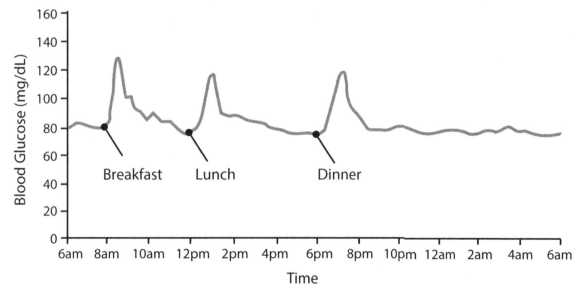

Figure 2.1. Typical Fluctuations in Plasma Glucose Over a Day

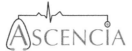

A **fasting plasma glucose (FPG)** test is drawn after patients have fasted for at least eight hours. It provides more precise information about normal circulating blood glucose levels, although other factors may still influence plasma glucose levels (e.g., stress or sleep patterns). An FPG is commonly used to assess for diabetes because it is easy to administer.

An **oral glucose tolerance test (OGTT)** is performed by having patients drink a solution containing a known amount of glucose (usually 75 grams). Their blood glucose is then tested two hours later. (Other intervals may be used.) An OGTT is usually used to diagnose gestational diabetes.

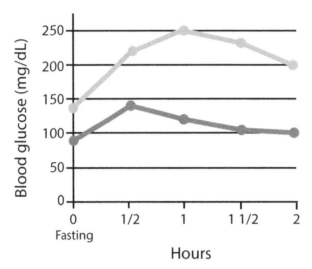

Figure 2.2. Plasma Glucose Levels During Oral Glucose Tolerance Test

Glucose in the blood will bond to hemoglobin in red blood cells, creating **glycated hemoglobin** (HbA1C, commonly known as **A1C**). An increased amount of circulating glucose will lead to an increased amount of A1C. The life span of a red blood cell is around three months, so A1C is a measurement of blood glucose levels over the previous three months. Because A1C shows an average of blood glucose over a long period of time, it is used to screen patients for diabetes and assess glycemic control in patients with diabetes.

> **Helpful Hint**:
>
> **C-peptide** is a protein produced by the beta cells of the pancreas during the production of insulin. C-peptide levels are used as a proxy to measure insulin production, particularly in people who are receiving exogenous insulin.

Table 2.4. Laboratory Tests for Plasma Glucose	
Test	**Normal Range**
random plasma glucose	<140 mg/dL
fasting plasma glucose (FPG)	70 – 100 mg/dL
2-hour oral glucose tolerance test (OGTT)	<140 mg/dL
hemoglobin A1C	<5.7%

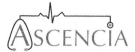

A1C is usually reported as the percentage of hemoglobin that is glycated. It can also be reported as **estimated average glucose (eAG)**, which is the blood glucose level, in mg/dL, that corresponds to A1C percentage. The eAG is found using the following formula:

- $eAG = (28.7 \times A1C) - 46.7$

Table 2.5. Converting Between A1C and eAG	
A1C (%)	**eAG (mg/dL)**
6	126
7	154
8	183
9	212
10	240
11	269
12	298

Practice Questions

20. How is a 2-hour 75 g OGTT administered?

21. An A1C test measures levels of which biological molecule?

22. What is the normal range for fasting plasma glucose?

23. What is the estimated average blood glucose of a person with an A1C of 8%?

Blood Glucose Monitoring

Blood glucose monitoring (BGM) determines blood glucose levels at the moment the test is performed. Blood glucose (BG) may be checked by patients at any time with a BGM device that requires patients to place a drop of blood on a **test strip**. The test strip contains an enzyme (either glucose oxidase or glucose dehydrogenase) that reacts with glucose, allowing the meter to determine the amount of glucose in the sample. Patients using a BGM device should follow these steps each time they check their BG:

1. Wash hands thoroughly with soap and dry well.

2. Put the test strip into the monitor.

3. Stick the middle or ring finger with the lancet; always stick on the side (not the center) of the fingertip (see Figure 2.3.).

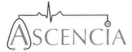

4. Place the blood droplet onto the strip and wait the allotted time (usually a few seconds) for a reading to appear.

lancet finger stick location

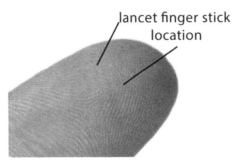

Figure 2.3. Finger Stick Location

Blood glucose monitoring is essential for patients who are taking insulin because it allows them to check for hypo- or hyperglycemia and adjust insulin doses as needed. Patients who require basal and bolus insulin or who use an insulin pump should check their BG levels at the following times:

- before eating (and after as necessary)
- at bedtime
- before exercising
- after treating hypoglycemia
- before critical tasks

The target BG level for adults is 80 – 130 mg/dL while fasting or before eating. For a 1- to 2-hour postprandial check, the target should be <180 mg/dL. The target is generally lower for children and people who are pregnant.

BGM is not required for people with diabetes (PWD) who take only basal insulin or antidiabetic agents; however, patients may benefit from periodic testing to better understand how their BG responds to specific foods, exercise, or other factors. It may also be required to assess hypoglycemia in at-risk patients. Patients using BGM devices should be educated on factors that may affect the device's accuracy:

- environmental factors (e.g., temperature, humidity, and altitude): Patients should be aware of the ranges for their particular devices.
- incorrect use of meter: The most common source of error is contaminated hands.
- the use of expired, damaged, or counterfeit test strips
- medications: Common over-the-counter (OTC) substances that can affect BGM readings include acetaminophen (which can lead to an incorrectly high reading) and ascorbic acid (vitamin C).

> **Helpful Hint:**
>
> Because the amount of blood used by a BGM device is so small, even tiny amounts of sugar left on the hands can affect the readings.

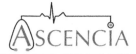
Practice Questions

24. What is the most common human error that leads to incorrect readings from a BGM device?

25. Where should a finger stick be done when testing BG?

26. What common OTC medications can affect readings from a BGM device?

Ketones

Diabetic ketoacidosis (DKA) happens when high levels of blood ketones develop when the liver converts fat to ketones, which makes the blood acidic. DKA is based on a triad of criteria that include the following:

- metabolic acidosis (serum bicarbonate < 15 mmol/l or venous pH < 7.3)

- ketonemia (> 3 mmol)

- and hyperglycemia (blood glucose > 11 mmol/l)

DKA is life-threatening and common in people with type 1 diabetes; it occurs due to infection, missed insulin shots, and stress from surgery. DKA occurs in patients with type 2 diabetes who experience surgical stress and who use SGLT-2 inhibitors. DKA management consists of four goals:

1. restoring circulating volume
2. correcting hyperglycemia through the reduction of plasma osmolarity and serum glucose
3. correcting electrolyte imbalance and hyperketonemia
4. identifying precipitating factors.

Hourly ketone levels and glucose levels must be monitored either by urine tests or blood glucose tests. Fluid and insulin therapy are the main elements of DKA management. DKA is resolved when ketone levels are less than 0.6 mmol/l and serum bicarbonate > 15 mmol/l.

Practice Question

27. What are the three main criteria that are used to diagnose DKA?

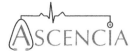

Weight and Weight Management

Obesity, particularly high levels of **visceral fat** (the fat that surrounds abdominal organs), is highly correlated with the development of type 2 diabetes. Current research supports the theory that excess fat surrounding muscle and liver cells prevents insulin from transporting glucose into these cells, leading to insulin resistance. Inflammation caused by obesity can also contribute to beta cell dysfunction.

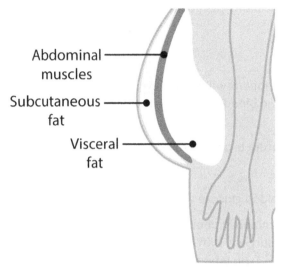

Figure 2.4. Visceral Fat in the Abdomen

Weight is classified using the **body mass index (BMI)**, a measurement of body fat that is based on a person's height and weight. To calculate the BMI, divide the weight in kilograms by the height in meters squared:

- $\text{BMI} = \frac{\text{kg}}{\text{m}^2}$

Patients with a BMI above 30 are classified as **obese**.

Table 2.6. BMI Scale	
<18.5	underweight
18.5 – 24.9	normal weight
25 – 29.9	overweight
30 – 34.9	obesity class I
35 – 39.9	obesity class II
>40	obesity class III

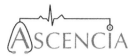

The BMI scale is based on data collected from White European populations, which can limit its usefulness in evaluating patients in other ethnic groups. For example, the BMI cutoff defining obesity (and diabetes risk) is lower for Asians and people of Asian descent because of differences in body composition.

There is also current scientific debate about the risks associated with high BMI for Americans of African descent, whom studies have shown are more likely to be overweight or obese. Some studies have shown their risk of developing diabetes to be comparable to that of White people with the same BMI; other studies have yielded mixed results, with some showing a higher risk for Americans of African descent and some showing a lower risk.

Weight loss is a key component of type 2 diabetes management. Studies have consistently shown health benefits for patients with type 2 diabetes who lose weight:

- improved glycemic control

- decreased blood pressure

- decreased lipid levels

- lower overall risk for CVD

- less need for medications to control blood glucose and CVD risk

> **Helpful Hint**:
>
> Obesity is a risk factor for developing diabetes and related complications, but weight alone does not determine how "healthy" a person is. A person who is overweight may never develop diabetes; conversely, a person who is considered to be of normal weight or underweight can be diagnosed with diabetes.

The benefits can be seen at weight losses of just 3 to 5% of body weight. Continued improvement may be seen as high weight loss goals are met. There are three options available to patients seeking to lose weight:

1. changes to dietary pattern and activity (discussed in detail in "Lifestyle Management")

2. medications (as described in Table 2.7.)

3. weight loss surgery

Table 2.7. FDA Approved Medications for Weight Loss	
Drug	**Description**
Orlistat	prevents absorption of fats; sold OTC as Alli
Phentermine/topiramate ER	combination CNS stimulant and appetite suppressant
Naltrexone/bupropion ER	combination opioid antagonist and antidepressant that suppress appetite
Liraglutide; semaglutide	type 2 diabetes medications that can increase weight loss

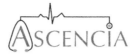

Practice Question

28. How is BMI calculated?

29. Which type of fat is associated with the development of type 2 diabetes?

30. A person with a BMI of 32 would fall into which category on the BMI scale?

31. Which two medications for type 2 diabetes are also recommended for weight loss?

Weight Loss Surgery

Bariatric surgery, also known as **metabolic surgery**, involves bypassing or removing sections of a patient's stomach. The procedure can lead to weight loss and improvements in glycemic control.

Evidence has indicated that bariatric surgery is more effective than medical therapy in regard to the treatment of type 2 diabetes and obesity. Bariatric surgery came about through the observation of how patients with upper gastrointestinal cancers underwent drastic weight loss when undergoing surgical resection. Medical professionals will inform patients with diabetes about how bariatric surgery procedures can be utilized for long-term weight loss. They will also make patients aware of any possible complications that can arise from existing chronic conditions. Types of bariatric surgery include

- sleeve gastrectomy,

- adjustable gastric banding,

- Roux-en-Y gastric bypass,

- one anastomosis gastric bypass, and

- biliopancreatic diversion/duodenal switch.

The selected procedure will depend on the individual's comorbidities, which can impact both physical and mental health. Patients who have had metabolic surgery should be advised to eat small, frequent meals and avoid liquids until 30 minutes after eating. They may also need to take vitamin and mineral supplements.

> **Helpful Hint**:
>
> **Dumping syndrome** is a collection of symptoms that result from rapid gastric emptying following bariatric surgery. It can cause postprandial hypoglycemia when the rapid delivery of carbohydrates into the intestines causes an overproduction of insulin.

Practice Questions

32. Which type of bariatric surgery is BEST for patients with diabetes who have a history of reflux?

Activity and Activity Management

Exercise may lower or raise blood glucose levels, depending on the length and intensity of activity. Generally, low- to medium-intensity activities will lower blood glucose levels by increasing insulin uptake in muscle cells. This effect may last up to eight hours. High-intensity activities, such as sprints and weightlifting, may cause a release in adrenaline, which raises blood glucose levels.

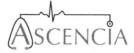

People with diabetes should be advised to closely monitor glucose levels before and after exercising to learn how their bodies respond to different types of activities. They may need to make adjustments to account for changes in blood glucose during and after exercise. Precautions may include

- decreasing the insulin dose before activity,

- increasing carbohydrate consumption before activity,

- keeping fast-acting glucose nearby while exercising, and

- not exercising during peak insulin action times.

Practice Question

33. Which type of exercise is likely to raise blood glucose levels?

Chapter 2 Answer Key

1. Diabetes is characterized by deficiencies in carbohydrate metabolism that result in hyperglycemia.

2. Diabetes is categorized based on the underlying etiology of the hyperglycemia.

3. During the waking process, the body releases cortisol and growth hormone, which raise blood glucose levels.

4. The three most common presenting symptoms of hyperglycemia are polyuria, polydipsia, and polyphagia.

5. A fasting plasma glucose of ≥126 mg/dL indicates diabetes.

6. An A1C of 6.5% indicates diabetes.

7. The presence of pancreatic autoantibodies and asymptomatic hyperglycemia is characteristic of stage 2 of type 1 diabetes.

8. A random plasma glucose of ≥200 mg/dL is sufficient to diagnose diabetes in patients with symptoms of hyperglycemia.

9. The range of A1C that indicates prediabetes is 5.7% – 6.4%.

10. Obesity with fat distributed around the abdomen is correlated to a higher risk for type 2 diabetes.

11. Patients may not realize they have these symptoms since they can develop gradually over many years.

12. According to ADA guidelines, a 38-year-old with no risk factors for diabetes should be screened for prediabetes every three years.

13. Type 2 diabetes is caused by decreasing insulin secretion from beta cells and insulin resistance.

14. Pregnant people should be screened for gestational diabetes at 24 – 28 weeks.

15. Hyperglycemia during pregnancy is linked to increased risk for preeclampsia, fetal abnormalities, preterm delivery, larger delivery weight, and cesarean section.

16. The underlying mechanisms that lead to gestational diabetes mellitus (GDM) are similar to those that cause type 2 diabetes, and people with GDM are at very high risk of developing type 2 diabetes later in life.

17. Monogenic diabetes is diagnosed through genetic testing.

18. The most common causes of pancreatic diabetes are cystic fibrosis, pancreatitis, hemochromatosis, and resection of pancreatic tissue.

19. Corticosteroids are the most common cause of drug-induced diabetes.

20. A 2-hour 75 g oral glucose tolerance test (OGTT) is administered by having patients drink 75 grams of glucose and measuring their plasma glucose two hours later.

21. An A1C test measures levels of glycated hemoglobin.

22. The normal range for fasting plasma glucose is 70 – 100 mg/dL.

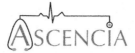

23. An A1C of 8% corresponds to an eAG of 183 mg/dL.

24. The most common human error that leads to incorrect readings from a blood glucose monitoring (BGM) device is contaminated hands.

25. The finger stick should be done on the side of the tip of the middle or ring finger.

26. Acetaminophen and vitamin C are over-the-counter (OTC) medications that can lead to incorrect readings from a blood glucose monitoring (BGM) device.

27. The diagnostic criteria for DKA include monitoring the plasma glucose concentration, plasma ketones, and either the pH, anion gap, or bicarbonate level.

28. Body mass index (BMI) is calculated by dividing the weight in kilograms by the height in meters squared: $BMI = \frac{kg}{m^2}$.

29. Visceral fat—which surrounds organs and is often located in the abdomen—is associated with the development of type 2 diabetes.

30. A person with a body mass index (BMI) of 32 would be considered obesity class I on the BMI scale.

31. Liraglutide and semaglutide are drugs that may help with weight loss.

32. Roux-en Y gastric bypass (RYGB) is considered a treatment for patients with reflux and obesity.

33. High-intensity activities, such as sprints and weightlifting, may raise blood glucose levels.

Chapter 3 – Self-Management Behaviors and Preferences

Eating and Activity Habits and Preferences

Medical Nutrition Therapy

Patients with diabetes should always be offered **medical nutrition therapy**—nutrition counseling from a registered dietician to help with the management of blood glucose levels and cardiovascular risk. Nutrition therapy for PWD should be individualized; there is not one specific dietary pattern recommended for glucose management, and there is no such thing as a "diabetes diet."

Instead of a one-size-fits-all approach, diabetes care and education specialists should focus on general guidelines that promote improved health outcomes and work to integrate these guidelines with the patient's tastes and lifestyle. Generally, a healthy dietary pattern should include the following components:

- fruits and non-starchy vegetables

- lean proteins

- whole grains

- unsaturated fats

- foods rich in fiber

- small amounts of refined grains and simple sugars

- small amounts of saturated fats and cholesterol

The American Diabetes Association (ADA) and the Academy of Nutrition and Dietetics recommend a number of different dietary patterns and meal-planning methods that can be adapted to individual patients to help manage type 2 diabetes. These include the plate method, the Mediterranean-style diet pattern, low carbohydrate dietary patterns, low fat dietary patterns, and the DASH diet.

The **plate method** provided by the ADA can help patients who have difficulty counting, weighing, or measuring foods. The plate method divides the plate so that the meal consists of one-half non-starchy vegetables, one-quarter

> **Helpful Hint**:
>
> **Fad diets** can be challenging to adhere to, boring, and nutritionally inadequate. Most people will also gain back any weight lost while on a fad diet. Patients who want to lose weight should be encouraged to develop a healthy, sustainable dietary pattern.

> **Helpful Hint**
>
> Shelf-stable, budget-friendly foods that can be recommended for patients managing type 2 diabetes include lower sodium canned beans, canned tuna, and tomato products; peanut butter with no added sugar; unsweetened canned fruit; and oatmeal.

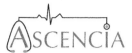

carbohydrates, and one-quarter protein. It also includes water or another zero-calorie drink.

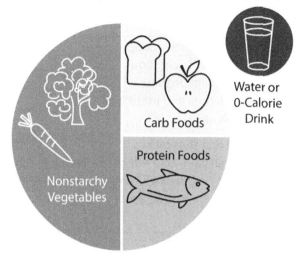

Figure 3.1. The ADA Plate Method

The **Mediterranean style** of eating is based on the cultures of Greece and Italy. It focuses on whole grains, beans and other legumes, vegetables, fruits, and nuts. The main source of fat in this dietary pattern is olive oil, and the main sources of protein are fish and legumes. Red meat and desserts are rarely eaten. Controlled studies have shown that a Mediterranean-style dietary pattern can reduce blood glucose and the need for antidiabetic agents.

A **low- or very low-carbohydrate dietary pattern** limits carbohydrate intake. These dietary patterns can be helpful in lowering blood glucose, but patients often need to set a very low limit (less than 26% of calories from carbohydrates) to see results. A **low-fat** style of eating may help patients lose weight but is generally not useful for lowering blood glucose levels.

The **Dietary Approaches to Stop Hypertension (DASH) diet** is often suggested to patients as part of a comprehensive plan to lower blood pressure. The DASH diet shares many features with the general guidelines described above, including a focus on whole grains, non-starchy vegetables and limiting saturated fat.

The main feature of the DASH diet is a limit on daily sodium intake to under 2,300 milligrams (or less for people struggling to control their blood pressure). This dietary pattern also promotes consumption of foods high in potassium, calcium, and magnesium, which may also help reduce blood pressure.

Patients may have special considerations that could impact their dietary patterns and meal planning. Some of these are summarized in Table 3.1.

Table 3.1. Special Considerations for Meal Planning		
Consideration	**Description**	**Education and Meal Planning**
Alcohol consumption	prevents the liver from releasing glucose for up to 12 hours, resulting in hypoglycemia; can interact with sulfonylureas, causing hypoglycemia	People with diabetes who take insulin or antidiabetic agents should always eat carbohydrates when drinking alcohol, particularly before going to bed.

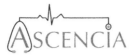

Table 3.1. Special Considerations for Meal Planning		
Consideration	**Description**	**Education and Meal Planning**
Food insecurity	the lack of regular access to enough food, either from insufficient food purchasing power or inadequate access to the appliances and utensils necessary for cooking	Specialists should be ready to recommend cheaper, shelf-stable options to these patients to help them stick to their care plan.
Gastroparesis	slow gastric emptying that causes bloating, abdominal pain, acid reflux, or nausea and vomiting; hypoglycemia that can result from slow or delayed meal absorption	Eating five to six small meals a day that are lower in fiber and fat helps with digestion.
Celiac disease	an autoimmune condition that causes intolerance to gluten protein in wheat, rye, barley, and some oats; causes diarrhea, malabsorption, and anemia	People with celiac disease should follow a completely gluten-free dietary pattern.

Helpful Hint:

Dietary lifestyle interventions should be developmentally and culturally appropriate for children and adolescents with diabetes. The specialist should recognize that peers will influence the likelihood of a patient's adherence to lifestyle changes.

Practice Questions

1. Which type of food takes up the largest portion of the plate in the ADA's plate method?

2. What are the main sources of protein in the Mediterranean-style dietary pattern?

3. What is the maximum amount of daily sodium allowed on the DASH diet?

4. What will happen to the blood glucose level of a patient with type 1 diabetes who skips dinner and has two glasses of wine before bed?

5. Which protein should patients with celiac disease avoid entirely?

Activity Habits and Preferences

To improve health, people with diabetes should be encouraged to engage in **physical activity**. Regular exercise has many proven health benefits:

- reduced A1C
- lowered insulin resistance

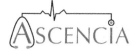

- lower blood pressure and lipid levels

- lower overall risk for CVD

The American College of Sports Medicine (ACSM) recommends a mix of aerobic activity and resistance training. A summary of their recommendations is described in Table 3.2.

Table 3.2. ACSM Exercise Recommendations	
Type of Exercise	**Per Week**
aerobic (moderate)	150 minutes minimum
aerobic (vigorous/interval training)	75 minutes
resistance (muscle strengthening)	2 – 3 sessions with at least one day between sessions
flexibility and balance training	2 – 3 times a week for older adults

Helpful Hint:

The ACSM recommends that all children get sixty minutes a day or more of moderate to vigorous activity.

Practice Question

6. How many minutes of moderate aerobic activity does the ACSM recommend people with diabetes get every week?

Medication Practices and Preferences

Diabetes care and education specialists should understand the fundamentals of pharmacology, including drug actions and adverse reactions. This knowledge will allow specialists to help patients find the antidiabetic agent that works best for their health and lifestyle.

The majority of **drugs** act by mimicking or suppressing normal physiological processes in the body. Drugs cannot change the fundamental physiological processes that occur in the body—they can only change the rate at which they occur. Drug action occurs when the drug binds to receptors on a protein molecule in the body to activate or block a physiological process:

- An **agonist** binds to receptors and stimulates activity.

  - For example, nitroglycerin is an agonist that results in the activation of enzymes that dilate blood vessels.

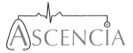

- Endogenous agonists (e.g., serotonin, epinephrine) are the molecules produced by the body that naturally bind to receptor sites.
- An **antagonist** binds to a receptor to block activity.

  - For example, ACE inhibitors block the angiotensin-converting enzyme (ACE), which normally causes blood vessels to constrict. The result is dilation of the blood vessels.

Practice Question

7. How does an agonist activate a physiological process?

Prescription Drugs, Antidiabetic Agents, and Adverse Reactions

The **brand name** of a drug is the name it is given by the pharmaceutical company that funded its research and development. This company holds the drug's patent for up to twenty years after its initial development, but when the patent expires, other pharmaceutical companies can produce the drug.

A **generic drug** must have the same active ingredient, strength, and dosage form as the brand-name drug, but the inactive ingredients do not need to be the same. Many generic drugs cost less to produce because generic manufacturers do not need to recoup the cost of research and development.

> **Helpful Hint**:
> Therapeutic equivalent/generic drugs do not need to have the same appearance, packaging, preservatives, or flavor.

For the FDA to approve a generic drug, it must be therapeutically equivalent to the brand-name version, meaning it produces the same clinical effect and has the same safety profile. Generally, generic drugs can be substituted for prescribed brand-name medications (and vice versa) when the substitution will save the patient money. In fact, many insurers and state regulations require this substitution.

Type 2 diabetes can be treated with a variety of prescription antidiabetic agents that change how insulin is produced and used in the body:

- metformin
- DPP-IV inhibitors (gliptins)
- thiazolidinediones (TZDs)
- sulfonylureas (insulin secretagogues)
- meglitinides
- gemfibrozil (alpha-glucosidase inhibitors)
- SGLT2 inhibitors
- GLP-1 agonists
- amylin analogs (pramlintide)

The mechanism of action, administration, side effects, interactions, and warnings for each class of antidiabetic agents is discussed below in "Details of Antidiabetic Agents."

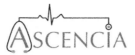

Metformin is the first-line therapy for almost all patients with T2D. For patients needing further BG control, other antidiabetic agents are added based on the patient's clinical characteristics. The most important factors to consider when selecting second-line antidiabetic agents are the presence of atherosclerotic cardiovascular disease (ASCVD), heart failure (HF), or chronic kidney disease (CKD):

- For patients with ASCVD, a glucagon-like peptide-1 (GLP-1) agonist with proven cardiovascular benefit is recommended.

- For patients with HF or CKD, a sodium-glucose cotransporter-2 (SGLT2) inhibitor with evidence of reducing HF or CKD is recommended if kidney function is adequate.

- In the absence of ASCVD, HF, or CKD, a GLP-1 agonist, SGLT2 inhibitor, DPP-IV inhibitor, or TZDs may be added.

Patients with T2D may also require insulin as the disease progresses. These patients are typically started on a basal insulin at 0.1 – 0.2 units/kg per day. Bolus insulin may be added if glycemic targets are not met. Indicators for insulin use in patients with T2D include the following:

- A1C >10%,

- BG ≥300 mg/dL

- symptoms of hyperglycemia

Allergic reactions of insulin were originally common due to impurities, such as pig or cow proteins and other additives or preservatives. The use of human and analog recombinant insulin has decreased insulin allergy to less than 1% of those administering insulin. Allergic reactions are categorized into general, immediate-local, and delayed/biphasic. **Delayed hypersensitivity allergic reactions** are the most common and appear about two weeks after initiating insulin therapy. Patients who use insulin pumps for subcutaneous insulin

> **Helpful Hint**:
>
> To minimize GI side effects of metformin, dosing can be increased by 500 mg increments every 4 – 8 weeks (depending on the patient).

delivery can have local infections at the site of needle insertion; patients must consider contact allergies due to the tape and tubing material. The adhesive patch on the skin can cause eczematous changes up to 11% in patients with diabetes. Patch testing is an important investigative tool for determining contact allergies.

Practice Questions

8. When choosing second-line antidiabetic agents to treat patients with type 2 diabetes, what are the most important factors to consider?

9. What characteristics must be shared between a brand-name drug and a generic equivalent?

10. What is the first-line drug for patients with T2D who require antidiabetic agents to control their BG levels?

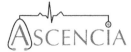

Details of Antidiabetic Agents

Metformin

Brand Names
Glucophage, Glumetza

Mechanism of Action

- Reduces glucose production from the liver

- Increases uptake and glucose utilization in the periphery

Dosing and Administration

- Initial: 500 mg orally once daily with the largest meal of the day

- Optimal dose: 1 g orally twice daily or 2 g orally once daily with the largest meal(s)

Common Side Effects
Gastrointestinal (GI) symptoms, including nausea, vomiting, diarrhea

ADRs and Warnings
Contraindicated in patients with lactic acidosis, DKA, and severe renal dysfunction
Can cause vitamin B12 deficiency

Interactions
Patients should:

- Limit alcohol use due to increased risk for lactic acidosis;

- Avoid concomitant use of cimetidine (Tagamet), lamotrigine (Lamictal), trimethoprim, and dolutegravir; and

- Hold metformin 48 – 72 hours prior to taking any iodinated or radiopaque contrast agents.

DPP-IV Inhibitors (Gliptins)

Brand Names

- Januvia (sitagliptin)

- Tradjenta (linagliptin)

- Onglyza (saxagliptin)

Mechanism of Action

- Potentiate the effects of incretin hormones, which regulate glucose homeostasis

- Suppress glucagon secretion, slow GI emptying, and reduce overall food intake by regulating appetite

Dosing and Administration

- Taken orally once daily with or without food

- DPP-IV inhibitors (except for linagliptin) require dose adjustment if renal function is low.

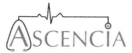

Common Side Effects

- Nasopharyngitis

- ermatologic reactions; usually benign maculopapular rash

- Stevens-Johnson syndrome or toxic epidermal necrolysis (potentially life-threatening)

ADR and Warnings

Data is conflicting, but DPP-IV inhibitor use has been linked to

- Arthralgias

- Pancreatitis

- Exacerbation of heart failure

> **Helpful Hint**
>
> Stevens-Johnson syndrome is characterized by flu-like symptoms and a blistering rash on the skin and mucous membranes.

Interactions

- Patients should avoid taking carbamazepine, rifampin, phenytoin, efavirenz, and St. John's wort with linagliptin.

- Saxagliptin dose may require adjustment if patients are taking any of the following: clarithromycin, erythromycin, diltiazem, itraconazole, ketoconazole, ritonavir, verapamil, and grapefruit juice.

- Patients should avoid a combination of GLP-1 therapy and DPP-IV inhibitors because there is an additive risk for pancreatitis.

Thiazolidinediones (TZDs)

Brand Names

- Actos (pioglitazone)

- Avandia (rosiglitazone)

Mechanism of Action

- Increase peripheral muscle glucose uptake and utilization

- Reduce glucose output from the liver

Administration
Taken orally once daily with or without food

Common Side Effects
Edema
Can worsen heart failure

ADRs and Warnings

- Rosiglitazone: boxed warning for fatal myocardial infarction

- Contraindicated in patients with NYHA class III – IV heart failure

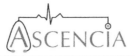

- Can be used by patients with NYHA I – II heart failure, but they must be monitored closely for rapid weight gain and dyspnea associated with bladder carcinoma risk; contraindicated in patients with a history of bladder cancer linked to acute hepatic failure and bone fractures

Interactions

Oral contraceptives and progestins interact with TZDs, resulting in possible loss of contraception.

Sulfonylureas (Insulin Secretagogues)

Brand Names

- Micronase, Glynase, DiaBeta (glyburide)

- Glucotrol (glipizide)

- Amaryl (glimepiride)

Mechanism of Action

Stimulate the pancreas to make and release insulin

Administration

Taken orally first thing in the morning about a half hour before breakfast can be taken with food if it causes stomach upset

Common Side Effects

- Nausea and vomiting

- Weight gain

ADRs and Warnings

- Per package labeling, use is contraindicated in patients with a sulfonamide allergy; however, the claim has been contested, and sulfonylureas can be used in this population with caution.

- Sulfonylureas may cause photosensitivity; skin protection is advised.

- The risk for hypoglycemia is elevated in older adults who skip meals and exercise vigorously.

- Glyburide and glimepiride are on the Beers list and should be avoided in patients who are 65 years and older.

Interactions

- Alcohol use should be limited.

- Concomitant insulin use should be avoided.

- Dose may need to be lowered with concomitant use of GLP-1 agonists or DPP-IV inhibitors.

Meglitinides

Brand Names

- Starlix (nateglinide)

- Prandin (repaglinide)

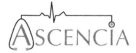

Mechanism of Action
Work similarly to sulfonylureas, except short-acting

Administration
Taken orally about a half hour before meals, 3 times a day; should be skipped if meal is skipped

Common Side Effects

- GI disturbances

- Headache

- Weight gain

ADRs and Warnings
Should be used with caution in patients with kidney and liver impairment

Interactions

- Alcohol use should be limited.

- NPH insulin is contraindicated with repaglinide due to myocardial infarction risk.

Gemfibrozil (Alpha-Glucosidase Inhibitors)

Brand Names

- Precose (acarbose)

- Glyset (miglitol)

Mechanism of Action

- Block digestive enzymes at brush border of the small intestines within the GI tract

- Decrease the rate of digestion of complex carbohydrates

- Reduce the absorption of glucose

Administration
Taken orally with the first bite of each meal, generally 3 times a day; should be skipped if meal is skipped

Common Side Effects
GI symptoms such as abdominal pain, diarrhea, flatulence, and bloating

ADRs and Warnings
Contraindicated in patients with history of cirrhosis, diabetic ketoacidosis, colonic ulceration, inflammatory bowel disease, or any intestinal disease that would affect absorption; contraindicated in patients who either have an intestinal obstruction or are at high risk for developing one

Serum creatinine >2

Interactions
Not systemically absorbed, does not have any clinically significant drug interactions

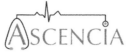

SGLT2 Inhibitors

<u>Brand Names</u>

- Invokana (canagliflozin)
- Farxiga (dapagliflozin)
- Jardiance (empagliflozin)
- Steglatro (ertugliflozin)

<u>Mechanism of Action</u>

- Inhibit sodium-glucose transporter-2, which is expressed in the proximal tubules in the kidney
- Less glucose reabsorbed into the blood
- More glucose excreted in the urine

<u>Administration</u>
Taken orally around the same time each day

<u>Common Side Effects</u>

- UTI, genital mycotic infections: Patients should thoroughly wipe and clean the urogenital area.
- Increased urination: Patients should stay hydrated to avoid hypovolemia.

<u>ADRs and Warnings</u>

- Contraindicated in patients with an estimated glomerular filtration rate <30 or who have end-stage renal disease
- Associated with increased risk for lower limb amputations (especially Invokana)
- Should be avoided in patients who have a greater risk for foot amputation, such as the presence of neuropathy, foot deformity, vascular disease, or history of foot ulceration
- Increased risk for hyperkalemia
- Nasopharyngitis (with dapagliflozin)
- Increased LDL (with empagliflozin)

<u>Interactions</u>

- Hypotension if patients are on concomitant ACE inhibitors or diuretic therapy
- May alter digoxin levels
- Caution with human UDP-glucuronosyltransferase (UGT) enzyme inducers (rifampin, ritonavir, phenytoin, phenobarbital)

GLP-1 Agonists

<u>Brand Names</u>

- Byetta (exenatide IR)
- Bydureon (exenatide XR)

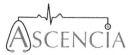

- Victoza (liraglutide)

- Ozempic, Rybelsus (semaglutide)

- Trulicity (dulaglutide)

Mechanism of Action

- Mimic enhancement of glucose-dependent insulin secretion

- Potentiate anti-hyperglycemic effects of incretin hormones

- Suppress glucagon secretion, slow gastric emptying, reduce food intake, and promote beta cell proliferation (the pancreatic cells responsible for manufacturing/secreting insulin)

Administration

- Irrespective of meals

- Oral, once daily: Rybelsus

- Injection, once daily: Victoza

- Injection, twice daily: Byetta

- Injections, once weekly: Bydureon, Ozempic, Trulicity

Common Side Effects
GI symptoms such as dyspepsia, nausea, vomiting, and diarrhea

ADRs and Warnings

- GLP-1 agonists are contraindicated in patients with a history of or active thyroid C-cell tumor (except for Byetta), severe GI disease such as Crohn's, obstruction, inflammatory bowel disease, ulcerative colitis, and gastroparesis.

- Byetta and Bydureon are contraindicated in patients with significant renal impairment (creatinine clearance of <30 ml/min).

- GLP-1 agonists are contraindicated in patients with pancreatitis.

- If pancreatitis (sudden abdominal pain along with nausea and vomiting) is suspected, GLP-1 therapy should be discontinued.

Interactions
The absorption of concomitantly administered oral medications can be delayed due to slowed gastric emptying.

Amylin Analogs (Pramlintide)

Brand Names
Symlin

Mechanism of Action

- Helps regulate postprandial hyperglycemia

- Slows gastric emptying and helps regulate appetite via central modulation

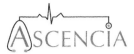

Administration
Injected subcutaneously immediately prior to meals; should be skipped if meal is skipped

Common Side Effects

- Well-tolerated

- Nausea, vomiting, and headache

ADRs and Warnings
Boxed warning for severe hypoglycemia:

- Typically seen within 3 hours of injection

- Highest risk in patients who are also taking insulin or who have type 1 diabetes

Interactions
Insulin and Symlin can be coadministered with close monitoring of BG levels and the appropriate dose reduction of Symlin.

Symlin should be avoided with strong anticholinergics (i.e., atropine, scopolamine, oxybutynin, clozapine), which can lead to clinically significant gastroparesis.

Adverse drug reaction (ADR) is a broad term used to describe unwanted, uncomfortable, or dangerous effects that result from taking a specific medication. Most adverse drug reactions are dose-related, but they can also be caused by allergic reactions or **idiosyncratic** (unexpected responses that are neither dose-related nor allergic) reactions. Adverse drug reactions are classified into six types, as described in Table 3.3.

> **Helpful Hint**
>
> Prescribing information, including dosage and side effects, about available drugs is compiled in the *Prescribers' Digital Reference* (formerly the *Physicians' Desk Reference*), also known as the PDR. This information is available online at http://www.pdr.net/ and is integrated into many health record systems.

Table 3.3. Types of Adverse Drug Reactions

Type	Description	Example
A: augmented	predictable reactions arising from the pharmacological effects of the drug; dependent on dose	hypoglycemia due to insulin
B: bizarre	unpredictable reactions; independent of dose	hypersensitivity (anaphylaxis) to penicillin
C: chronic	reactions caused by the cumulative dose (the dose taken over a long period of time)	osteoporosis with oral steroids

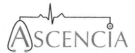

Table 3.3. Types of Adverse Drug Reactions		
Type	**Description**	**Example**
D: delayed	reactions that occur after the drug is no longer being taken	teratogenic effects with anticonvulsants
E: end-of-use	reactions caused by withdrawal from a drug	withdrawal syndrome with benzodiazepines
F: failure	unexpected failure of the drug to work; often caused by dose or drug interactions	resistance to antimicrobials

Practice Questions

11. What type of antidiabetic agent is likely to be prescribed to patients with T2D and moderate ASCVD who take metformin but are not meeting their glycemic target?

12. Should metformin be taken with or without food?

13. What are the most common side effects of SGLT2 inhibitors?

14. How should patients adjust their administration of Starlix if they plan to skip a meal?

15. Which antidiabetic agent has a boxed warning for fatal myocardial infarction?

16. Which non-insulin antidiabetic agents are associated with a higher risk for causing hypoglycemia?

17. A patient reports diarrhea on the second day of taking antibiotics. What type of adverse drug reaction is this?

18. Why should a patient avoid taking cimetidine while on metformin?

Nonprescription Medications and Antidiabetic Agents

People with diabetes should be aware that some medications may affect their BG levels or interact with their antidiabetic agents. Tables 3.4. and 3.5. discuss some of the most important drugs for patients to avoid or use with caution.

Table 3.4. Drug Interactions	
Antidiabetic Agent	**OTC Drug or Supplement**
Pramlintide (Symlin)	Avoid strong **anticholinergics** due to additive risk for gastroparesis, including first-generation antihistamines used for allergies or insomnia

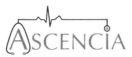

Table 3.4. Drug Interactions	
Antidiabetic Agent	**OTC Drug or Supplement**
	(diphenhydramine [Benadryl] and hydroxyzine [Vistaril]) and oxybutynin patch (Oxytrol) used for overactive bladder in women.
Linagliptin (Tradjenta)	**St. John's wort** (OTC supplement used for its antidepressant activity) can significantly reduce the effects of linagliptin.
Metformin	Avoid **cimetidine (Tagamet)**, which is an acid reducer that raises the concentration of metformin in the blood, increasing the risk for lactic acidosis.

Table 3.5. OTC Drugs and Supplements That Affect BG Levels	
OTC Medication or Supplement	**Effect on BG**
NSAIDs (e.g., ibuprofen, aspirin)	NSAIDs induce hypoglycemia, especially in those taking sulfonylureas. The effect is usually minor, but patients should be aware that their glucose levels can drop.
Oral decongestants (e.g., (pseudoephedrine and phenylephrine)	These raise BG levels by blocking insulin secretion and peripheral uptake of glucose into the cells and promoting glycogenolysis.
Niacin (vitamin B3)	This can cause hyperglycemia.
Alcohol (as an inactive ingredient)	In liquid formulations, alcohol can interact with a patient's sulfonylurea or insulin and increase the risk for hypoglycemia.
Carbohydrates (as inactive ingredients)	Carbohydrates can cause hyperglycemia; choose sugar-free versions of foods when available.

Practice Questions

19. How do oral decongestants raise blood glucose levels?

20. What OTC medications should patients avoid if they are taking Symlin?

21. What should be cautioned in a PWD who wants to use ibuprofen to treat a headache and fever?

22. What OTC medications or supplements may cause hyperglycemia?

Complementary and Alternative Medicines

Patients may look to OTC drugs, vitamins, minerals, or supplements to help manage their glucose levels. Although some of these will have little or no impact on glucose levels or diabetes symptoms, research

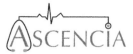

suggests that some of these supplements may be beneficial. The most popular vitamins and supplements are summarized in Table 3.6.

Table 3.6. OTC Vitamins and Other Supplements	
Alpha-lipoic acid	Doses between 600 and 1800 mg once daily appear to lessen neuropathy-related symptoms in people with diabetes.
Benfotiamine	This is converted to thiamine (vitamin B1) in the body and has established antioxidant effects; patients taking 600 mg in divided doses had reduced symptoms of diabetic neuropathy.
Cassia cinnamon	This may be effective for reducing FBG, with the recommended cinnamon dose ranging from 120 mg – 6 g daily.
Chromium	This is possibly effective in lowering FBG, insulin levels, PPG, and A1C; effects are more likely seen with doses >200 mcg, especially in patients with poorly controlled diabetes (A1C greater than 8%).
Coenzyme Q	This can lessen neuropathic symptoms in people with diabetes but has not been shown to be effective in glycemic control.
Fenugreek	This may reduce FBG, PPG, and A1C.
Flaxseed	Both whole and ground flaxseed have been shown to slightly lower A1C levels and modestly reduce FBG and insulin levels.
Garlic	Up to 1500 mg daily has been shown to lower FBG when taken alone or in combination with metformin for at least 12 weeks.
Probiotics	There is insufficient evidence to support its use with the intent to lower glucose levels or A1C in people with diabetes.
Psyllium husk	The FDA issued a qualified health claim stating that "psyllium husk may reduce the risk of type 2 diabetes," despite also concluding that there is insufficient evidence to support the claim.
Turmeric, ginger	More research is needed to establish their roles in blood glucose management.

Helpful Hint:

Decongestants delivered via nasal spray, such as oxymetazoline (e.g., Afrin), have less systemic exposure and are therefore less likely to affect glucose levels.

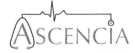

Practice Question

23. What is the maximum daily amount of garlic that has been shown to lower fasting blood glucose levels after 12 weeks?

Technology for Diabetes Self-Management

Monitors

Continuous glucose monitors (CGMs) work via a sensor placed under the skin. The sensor measures **interstitial glucose**—the amount of glucose in the fluid around cells. The level of interstitial glucose is not equal to BG levels; however, the levels of glucose in blood and in interstitial fluid are correlated, allowing the device to extrapolate BG levels.

There are three types of CGMs available:

- **Real-time (rtCGMs)** measure glucose levels at regular intervals (usually every 1 – 15 minutes) and transmit the data to a receiver. These devices may also have an alarm for hypo- and hyperglycemia.

- **Intermittently scanned CGMs (isCGMs)** require the user to hold a reader over the sensor to see a glucose readout.

- **Professional CGMs (P-CGMs)** are put in place by a provider and are usually worn for 10 – 14 days. These devices provide clinicians with data on BG trends for a specific patient.

> **Helpful Hint**:
>
> CGMs are meant to identify trends in glucose levels and should not be used to measure current BG levels. A BGM device should be used to check BG levels before making treatment decisions (e.g., adjusting an insulin dose).

All CGM devices transmit data to a receiver, such as a smartphone. The device's app will then allow users to see various metrics and trends designed to help them manage their BG levels. Metrics collected from CGMs and standard targets are summarized in Table 3.7. (Note that targets are for adult PWD with no comorbidities.)

> **Helpful Hint**
>
> During patient education, it is helpful to link new information to current behavior; new learning is better received when it focuses on what the patient already knows.

Table 3.7. Continuous Glucose Monitoring Metrics

Metric	Description	Target*
Time in range (TIR)	the amount of time spent in the target glucose range	70% of time at 70 – 180 mg/dL
Time above range (TAR)	the amount of time spent above the target glucose range	<25% of time above 180 mg/dL

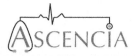
Metric	Description	Target*
		<5% of time above 250 mg/dL
Time below range (TBR)	the amount of time spent below the target glucose range	<4% of time below 70 mg/dL
		<1% of time below 54 mg/dL
Glucose management indicator (GMI)	an estimated A1C derived from 10 – 14 days of CGM data	<7%
Mean/average glucose	the average glucose value over a given time period	<154 mg/dL
Glycemic variability (% coefficient of variation [CV])	a measure of how often and how widely BG levels fluctuate	<33%

Table 3.7. Continuous Glucose Monitoring Metrics

*Targets are adapted from general ADA guidelines. Specialists should work with clinicians and patients to develop targets adapted to each individual patient.

CGM is becoming the standard for adult patients with type 1 diabetes (T1D); however, its usefulness for patients with type 2 diabetes (T2D) is still under review. As with BGM, the use of CGM is most impactful for patients taking basal and bolus insulin, though it may be appropriate for any PWD who are struggling with glycemic control. Potential downsides to CGM include contact dermatitis and cost, which is usually higher than traditional BGM devices.

Practice Questions

24. What do CGMs measure?

25. How is an intermittently scanned CGM different from a real-time CGM?

26. What is the standard TIR target for most PWD?

Online Education and Patient Portals

Specialists should also make use of technology to engage patients and connect them to providers and support communities. Many patients—particularly younger ones—are likely already online looking for health information. Specialists can use this enthusiasm to direct patients toward high-quality online resources:

- **Webinars** or streamed events are often available in the community and are geared toward specific patient populations, such as parents.

> **Helpful Hint**:
>
> An important part of integrating technology into an education plan is ensuring that patients can differentiate between good and bad sources of online health information.

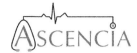

- Patients can often find support groups for specific conditions on **social media**. Specialists should caution patients to join such groups for *support*, <u>not</u> medical advice.

- Specialists should instruct patients on how to use **patient care interfaces** if they are available. These allow patients to send secure messages to providers and receive timely replies to questions.

Practice Question

27. What precautionary measure should specialists share with patients when encouraging them to join online support groups through social media?

Community Support Resources

Managing diabetes is a lot of work, and patients should never manage their care alone. Many patients will reach out to family and friends for help, but it can also be beneficial to seek out additional emotional and material support in the community. Important community support resources include care managers, case managers, social workers, and support groups.

Care managers, case managers, and social workers can all play an integral role in providing community support to PWD. **Care managers** coordinate with doctors, nurses, and other providers to create a cohesive care plan that meets the unique needs of a patient. **Case managers** have a broader range of responsibilities: depending on their qualifications and roles, they can help develop care plans and help with issues related to financing care, requesting accommodations in the workplace, and handling medical paperwork.

Social workers are involved in the community side of coordinating care. They can help PWD with tasks such as getting rides to appointments and finding ways to pay for care. They also help PWD and their families manage the emotional burdens of diabetes.

Support groups are an often-underutilized resource that can be extremely beneficial for PWD and their family members. These groups provide PWD the opportunity to find people who share their diagnosis. People in the group can express their negative feelings in a safe space, find friendships, and seek emotional support from others who understand the experience of living with diabetes.

Practice Questions

28. What is the purpose of a diabetes support group?

29. What does a care manager do?

Chapter 3 Answer Key

1. Non-starchy vegetables take up the largest portion of the plate—50%.

2. The main sources of protein in the Mediterranean-style dietary pattern are fish and legumes.

3. The DASH diet recommends a daily intake of no more than 2,300 milligrams of sodium. For people who struggle to control their blood pressure, the recommended daily sodium intake could be less than 2,300 milligrams.

4. This person will likely develop hypoglycemia.

5. Patients with celiac disease should avoid the protein gluten entirely.

6. The American College of Sports Medicine (ACSM) recommends 150 minutes of moderate aerobic activity every week.

7. The agonist binds to receptors and stimulates activity

8. The most important factors to consider when selecting second-line antidiabetic agents are the presence of atherosclerotic cardiovascular disease (ASCVD), heart failure (HF), or chronic kidney disease (CKD).

9. A generic equivalent drug must have the same active ingredient, strength, and dosage form as the brand-name drug, but the inactive ingredients do not need to be the same.

10. Metformin is a first-line drug for patients with type 2 diabetes (T2D).

11. A glucagon-like peptide-1 (GLP-1) agonist with proven cardiovascular benefit is recommended for patients with atherosclerotic cardiovascular disease (ASCVD) who require a second antidiabetic agent to control blood glucose.

12. To minimize GI upset, metformin should be taken orally with the largest meal of the day.

13. The most common side effects associated with sodium-glucose cotransporter-2 (SGLT2) inhibitor use are frequent urination, mycotic infections, and UTI.

14. If patients skip a meal, they should skip their dose of Starlix.

15. Rosiglitazone has a boxed warning for fatal myocardial infarction.

16. Sulfonylureas and meglitinides are associated with a higher risk for causing hypoglycemia.

17. Diarrhea from antibiotics is an augmented reaction, which means it is a predictable reaction resulting from the pharmacological effects of the drug.

18. Cimetidine (Tagamet) is an acid reducer that raises the concentration of metformin in the blood, increasing the risk for lactic acidosis; patients taking metformin should therefore avoid cimetidine.

19. Oral decongestants raise blood glucose levels by blocking insulin secretion and peripheral uptake of glucose into the cells and promoting glycogenolysis.

20. Patients taking Symlin should avoid first-generation antihistamines, such as diphenhydramine, and strong anticholinergics, such as oxybutynin patches, which are available over the counter.

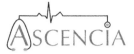

21. There is a risk for NSAIDs, such as ibuprofen, to induce hypoglycemia— especially in people with diabetes (PWD) who take sulfonylureas.

22. Some oral decongestants, such as pseudoephedrine and phenylephrine, and niacin (vitamin B3) may cause hyperglycemia.

23. Patients taking up to 1500 mg of garlic daily—alone or with metformin—have experienced lower fasting blood glucose after 12 weeks.

24. Continuous glucose monitors (CGMs) measure interstitial glucose—the amount of glucose in the fluid around cells.

25. An intermittently scanned continuous glucose monitor (CGM) only provides a reading when the reader is held over the scanner, while a real-time CGM automatically reads glucose levels at regular intervals.

26. The standard time in range (TIR) target for most patients with diabetes (PWD) is 70% of time at 70 – 180 mg/dL.

27. Specialists should always ensure that patients join such groups for support only—not for medical advice.

28. Support groups for people with diabetes allow individuals to find support from others who understand the experience of living with diabetes.

29. Care managers work with doctors, nurses, and other health care providers to coordinate care for patients and create unique care plans that fit an individual's needs.

Chapter 4 – Self-Management Skills and Learning

Self-Management Skills

In addition to basing their work on best practices, certified diabetes care and education specialists should lead by using the latest teaching techniques.

Specialists may work as part of a **diabetes self-management education and support (DSMES)** program. These programs are designed to teach patients the knowledge, skills, and abilities they need to self-manage diabetes. They also provide ongoing support so that self-management behaviors can be maintained throughout the patient's lifetime. There are five key points in time at which DSMES services should be provided to patients:

1. At diagnosis: All patients with newly diagnosed diabetes should be referred to a comprehensive DSMES program that addresses behavioral health and lifestyle modifications.

2. Annually: Patients should meet regularly with a specialist to review knowledge and skills.

3. When not meeting targets: More frequent intervention by specialists may be required if patients are not meeting self-management targets.

4. At development of complicating factors: Changes in health conditions (including pregnancy), physical limitations, and psychosocial factors should prompt referral of patients to DSMES.

The **ADCES7 self-care behaviors** (described in Table 4.1.) form the foundation for an effective and patient-centered DSMES program. The framework includes seven key principles that help patients change their behaviors and self-manage their diabetes. Patients should be educated on these principles as part of a DSMES program. The principles should also be used to guide health care team members as they work with the patient to develop a management plan.

Table 4.1. Summary of the ADCES7 Self-Care Behaviors	
Behavior	**Patient Goals**
1. Healthy coping	• developing a positive attitude toward diabetes and diabetes self-management • building self-sufficiency and resources for support
2. Healthy eating	• eating a variety of nutrient-rich foods to promote health • developing healthy eating patterns and personalized meal plans • being able to use nutrition labels

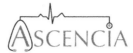

Table 4.1. Summary of the ADCES7 Self-Care Behaviors	
Behavior	**Patient Goals**
3. Being active	• engaging in a variety of physical movement that includes aerobic and resistance training • decreasing time spent sitting down
4. Taking medication	• following prescribed medication regimen • taking medications at the correct time, with the correct frequency, and in the right dosage
5. Monitoring	• collecting personal data related to other self-care behaviors and using this data to guide care decisions
6. Reducing risk	• identifying and mitigating risks for diabetes complications and comorbidities
7. Problem-solving	• being able to identify problems, develop possible solutions, and select the most effective courses of action • evaluating the success of problem-solving strategies

Practice Questions

1. What are the seven ADCES self-care behaviors?

2. What are the five situations in which patients should be offered DSMES services?

Learning-Related Objectives, Considerations, and Readiness

Patients' willingness and ability to learn depend on their motivation, readiness, functional status, and health literacy. The specialist should assess patients for each of these factors and build a plan that realistically reflects the individual patient's abilities and needs.

Motivation is the driving force behind people's actions. Specialists should work with patients to identify their sources of motivation and incorporate this knowledge into their education plans. People can be intrinsically or extrinsically motivated to achieve a goal:

- **Intrinsic motivation** is the desire to achieve a goal, seek challenges, or complete a task; it is driven by enjoyment and personal satisfaction (e.g., exercising because it is enjoyable).

- **Extrinsic motivation** is the desire to accomplish a goal; it is driven by external rewards or punishment (e.g., exercising to prevent cardiovascular disease).

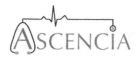

A patient's **functional status**—the ability to perform basic cognitive and physical tasks—will affect that person's ability to learn. Patients with **physical impairments** may lack the strength, coordination, and/or sensory abilities to learn new skills. **Cognitive impairments** may disrupt patients' abilities to process new knowledge and maintain emotional stability. Functional status can be measured by assessing patients' abilities to perform daily activities:

> **Helpful Hint**:
>
> Patients with an **external locus of control** will attribute their success or failure to outside forces. Patients with an **internal locus of control** will attribute their success or failure to themselves.

- **activities of daily living:** personal care activities such as toileting, bathing, dressing, and eating

- **instrumental activities of daily living:** more complex activities necessary for independent living, such as shopping and doing housework

Health literacy is the degree to which someone can find and understand basic health information needed to make personal health decisions. Patients' health literacy depends on many factors:

- communication skills and abilities

- cultural considerations

- knowledge of health topics

- situation or context of the information delivery

According to the US Department of Education's National Center for Education Statistics, populations that are vulnerable to poor health literacy include people aged over 65 years, minorities, people with mental illness, immigrants, and people with low incomes.

Specialists should assess patients' levels of health literacy when developing education plans. Health literacy assessments include the following:

- Rapid Estimate of Adult Literacy in Medicine (REALM)

- the Test of Functional Health Literacy in Adults (TOFHLA)

- the Newest Vital Sign (NVS) screening tool

> **Helpful Hint**:
>
> Part of diabetes education may require the specialist to "unteach" incorrect or oversimplified knowledge.

Specialists should develop a list of **learning objectives** based on their assessments of patients. This list should be prioritized based on the patients' preferences and health needs. The individualized education plans should also be sequenced in a manner that optimizes learning: concepts should flow from simple to complex, and lesson plans should build on previous learning.

Patient safety may require prioritizing initial teaching to include the recognition of symptoms and emergency management. For example, a first lesson plan might include a simple definition of diabetes and how to recognize and respond to hyper- and hypoglycemic emergencies. A subsequent lesson plan might include a discussion of the long-term side effects of hyperglycemia.

Readiness for behavior change describes people's drive to seek out new information and to incorporate that information into their lives. Patients' readiness to change can be shaped by many factors:

- openness to new information

- emotional response to illness (e.g., denial, anxiety)

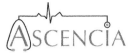

- religious and cultural beliefs

- social support systems

The specialist should assess a patient's readiness to change and then adapt the delivery of information to meet the patient's needs.

Table 4.2. Stages of Readiness for Change		
Stage	**Description**	**Specialist Goals**
Precontemplation	Patient is unaware of the problem or does not want to change.	Educate patient on issues and on the benefits of behavioral changes.
Contemplation	Patient is aware of the problem and thinking about making changes in the future.	Continue to provide education on issues and encourage patient to begin making a plan.
Preparation	Patient is making a plan to implement behavioral changes.	Help patient set S.M.A.R.T goals and develop a plan to meet those goals.
Action	The patient's plan has been implemented.	Help the patient implement the plan for behavioral change; provide support and assist with problem-solving.
Maintenance	Reinforcement is used to continue behavioral changes.	Reinforce behaviors with reminders and encouragement; provide support during setbacks and suggest adjustments to plan.

Practice Questions

3. A patient is setting an exercise goal and wants to buy something special when that goal is met. Is this intrinsic or extrinsic motivation?

4. A patient has been thinking about starting an exercise program but does not have time right now. In which stage of readiness to change is the patient, and how can the specialist encourage that behavioral change?

5. Which populations are statistically most vulnerable to poor health literacy?

Instructional Methods and Preferred Learning Styles

Instructional strategies should be chosen to address specific learning domains and learning styles. Psychologist Benjamin Bloom described three **domains of learning:**

- The **cognitive domain** (knowledge) includes collecting, synthesizing, and applying knowledge.

- The **affective domain** (attitude) involves emotions and attitudes, including the ability to be aware of emotions and respond to them.

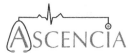

- The **psychomotor domain** (skills) relates to motor skills, including the ability to perform complex skills and create new movement patterns.

Helpful Hint:

During patient education, it is helpful to link new information to current behavior; new learning is better received when it focuses on what the patient already knows.

Education plans should address all three learning domains. For example, a patient who is learning about smoking cessation may need to be taught about the negative health impacts of smoking (cognitive domain), how to manage negative emotions related to quitting (affective domain), and how to correctly apply a nicotine patch (psychomotor domain).

Learning style is a person's preferred method of receiving new information. Most people do not learn best using a single style; instead, specialists should use multiple styles to reinforce knowledge:

- **Visual learning** can be accommodated with pictures, diagrams, and modeling.

- **Auditory learning** makes use of spoken language, mnemonic devices, and music.

- **Kinesthetic** (physical) **learning** focuses on bodily motion.

- **Social learning** employs interactions with other people.

- **Solitary learning** is accomplished alone.

Specialists who work with adult patients should be aware of the distinct traits of **adult learners**. Adults may learn more slowly than younger learners, be resistant to change, and require justification for new behaviors. On the other hand, adult learners can be more independent and self-directed than younger patients. Specialists should also keep in mind that older adults may struggle with technology more than "digital natives" and therefore require additional instruction to use technology, such as glucose monitoring with integrated apps.

The **instructional plan** should be tailored to the patient's learning objectives, developmental level, academic abilities, and preferred learning styles. Specialists may select from a wide range of instruction strategies when educating patients:

- **Lectures** (groups or one-on-one) are effective for conveying cognitive knowledge, particularly to auditory learners.

- **Group discussions** in which patients can ask questions are effective for social learners and can help with affective learning, such as changing attitudes.

- **Role-playing** is acting out a scenario involving interactions between people, such as family members, teachers, or health care providers. Role-playing is a good way to teach affective skills, such as responding to peer pressure.

- **Simulation** is acting out decisions and actions (rather than personal interactions, as in role-playing). For example, patients may simulate taking their blood glucose (BG) levels and deciding on actions to take based on specific readings.

- **Demonstrations** or **modeling** are useful for teaching psychomotor skills, such as checking blood glucose levels or administering insulin.

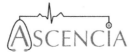

- **Instructional materials**, such as films or pamphlets, may be used as part of a larger education plan; however, they may be ineffective if patients are disengaged or the material does not match their needs and learning abilities.

Practice Questions

6. A specialist is teaching a patient how to take a blood pressure (BP) reading. While the patient is trying to apply the cuff, the specialist asks the patient to state the target BP range. The patient becomes visibly frustrated and claims to not know. How can the specialist adjust the teaching style to meet this patient's needs?

7. Which instructional strategy is MOST likely to be effective when teaching young patients how to discuss their diabetes diagnosis with teachers?

Chapter 4 Answer Key

1. The ADCES7 self-care behaviors are healthy coping, healthy eating, being active, taking medication, monitoring, reducing risk, and problem-solving.

2. Patients should be provided with diabetes self-management education and support (DSMES) services at diagnosis, annually, when they are not meeting targets, after the development of complicating factors, and during transitions in life and care.

3. The patient has extrinsic motivation: the desire to accomplish a goal that is driven by external rewards.

4. The patient is in the contemplation stage. The specialist can continue to provide education on physical activity and encourage the patient to begin making a plan.

5. According to the US Department of Education's National Center for Education Statistics, populations that are vulnerable to poor health literacy include people aged over 65 years, minorities, people with mental illness, immigrants, and people with low incomes.

6. The specialist disturbed the patient's focus on a psychomotor skill by asking about the blood pressure target. The specialist can help by focusing on one domain at a time: the patient should master the skills needed to take a blood pressure reading; then, the specialist can assess the patient's knowledge.

7. Role-playing (acting out a scenario involving interaction between people) is the strategy most likely to be effective when teaching communication skills, such as discussing a diabetes diagnosis.

Chapter 5 - Disease Process and Approach to Treatment

Diagnosis and Classifications

The Endocrine System

The endocrine system is made up of **endocrine glands** that secrete **hormones**—chemical messengers that travel through the bloodstream and regulate numerous body processes. These hormones regulate a wide variety of bodily processes, including metabolism; growth and development; sexual reproduction; the sleep-wake cycle; and hunger.

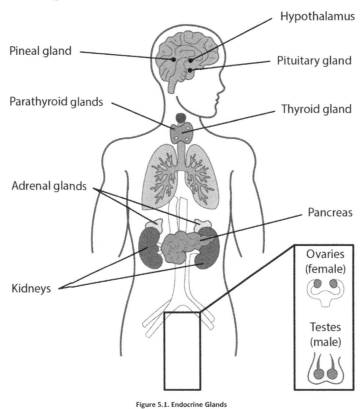

Figure 5.1. Endocrine Glands

Several endocrine glands play an integral role in the maintenance of blood sugar levels:

- The **pancreas** produces **insulin** and **glucagon** to balance blood sugar levels.
- The **thyroid** produces **thyroxine (T4)** and **triiodothyronine (T3)**, which regulate metabolism (energy use).

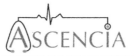

- The **adrenal glands** produce **epinephrine**, **norepinephrine**, and **cortisol**, which stimulate the fight-or-flight response.

- The **pituitary gland** produces **adrenocorticotropic hormone (ACTH)**, which stimulates the adrenal glands, and **somatotropin** (human growth hormone, or hGH), which regulates growth and metabolism.

- The **hypothalamus** receives input from the nervous system and regulates the pituitary gland.

Hormones can generally be described as either anabolic or catabolic:

- **Anabolic hormones** trigger processes that allow small molecules to bond together to create larger ones. For example, anabolic steroids stimulate cells to produce more proteins.

- **Catabolic hormones** stimulate cells to break down large molecules into smaller ones, releasing energy. Examples of catabolic hormones include cortisol and adrenaline, both of which promote the breakdown of large sugars into smaller ones that can be used by cells for energy.

Hormones are an important part of the human body's complex systems that maintain **homeostasis**—the body's internal equilibrium. These systems allow the body to monitor external changes and adapt by altering body temperature, blood sugar, blood pressure, and other physiological states.

Feedback mechanisms are the primary forms of communication between the systems working to maintain homeostasis. In a **negative feedback loop**, an external change prompts a response to return the body's internal environment to equilibrium. For example, if exposure to heat causes the body's internal temperature to rise, the body will attempt to cool down (a process called **thermoregulation**). Receptors in the skin detect the change in temperature and relay the message to the hypothalamus, which signals sweat glands to release sweat, cooling the body.

Practice Questions

1. Which endocrine gland secretes somatotropin?

2. Which type of cellular activity does anabolic hormones stimulate?

3. How does a negative feedback loop maintain homeostasis?

Glucose

Glucose Synthesis

Carbohydrates (sugars) are molecules made of carbon, hydrogen, and oxygen. Sugars are primarily used in organisms as a source of energy. They are **catabolized** (broken down) during cellular respiration to create molecules, such as adenosine triphosphate (ATP), that release energy that can then be used to drive cellular processes.

The main sugar used in cellular respiration is **glucose**. Glucose is a **monosaccharide**, a simple sugar that can bond together to form larger sugar molecules called **polysaccharides**. Animal cells store energy in

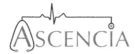

the form of the polysaccharide **glycogen**, which is built from glucose molecules during the process of **glycogenesis**. Glycogen is broken down into glucose during **glycogenolysis**.

Glucose: $C_6H_{12}O_6$

CH$_2$OH

O

OH

HO

OH

OH

Figure 5.2. Glucose

Glucose may also be stored as **lipids** (fats). During **lipogenesis**, glucose is converted to a fatty acid, which is transported to and stored in adipose tissue (body fat). Like glycogen, lipids can be broken down to provide energy for cells.

Practice Questions

4. What happens during glycogenesis?

5. What is glucose used for in the human body?

Glucose Homeostasis

Glucose homeostasis is the process that maintains the correct amount of glucose circulating in the blood, typically between 90 and 100 mg/dL. This process is a negative feedback loop controlled by two hormones, insulin and glucagon:

- **Insulin** is an anabolic hormone secreted by the pancreas. It promotes the uptake of glucose into cells where it can used for cellular respiration or stored as glycogen or fat.

- **Glucagon** is a catabolic hormone secreted by the pancreas that stimulates the breakdown of glycogen into glucose.

When blood glucose levels are high, beta cells in the pancreas secrete insulin. Insulin promotes glycogenesis (the storage of glucose as glycogen) in musculoskeletal, liver, and fat cells, which lowers blood glucose levels. When blood glucose levels are low, alpha cells in the pancreas secrete glucagon. Glucagon promotes glycogenolysis (the

Helpful Hint:

Insulin *lowers* blood glucose by stimulating the use and storage of glucose; glucagon *raises* blood glucose by stimulating the breakdown of glycogen into glucose.

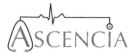

breakdown of glycogen into glucose) in the liver, which raises blood glucose levels.

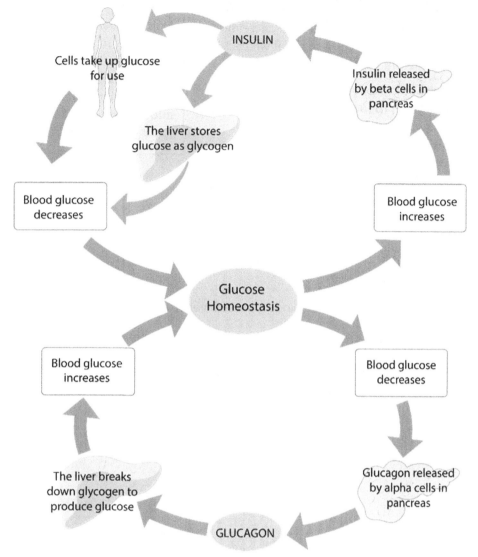

Figure 5.3. Glucose Homeostasis

Other hormones may affect glucose levels either by regulating the release of insulin or glucagon or by directly promoting glucose release or storage:

- **Amylin** is released with insulin; it inhibits glucagon release and slows the emptying of the stomach to create a feeling of satiety.

- **Somatostatin** regulates the production of both insulin and glucagon in the pancreas.

- **Epinephrine**, **norepinephrine**, and **cortisol** stimulate the breakdown of glycogen and raise blood glucose levels.

- **Thyroxine** and **triiodothyronine** stimulate the breakdown of glycogen and raise blood glucose levels.

- **Pancreatic polypeptide (PP)** regulates levels of glycogen in the liver.

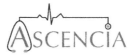

- Insulin, glucagon, and other hormones are produced in **pancreatic islets** (also called islets of Langerhans) distributed throughout the **pancreas**. Pancreatic islets contain five types of cells, each of which produces a different hormone:

    o **Alpha cells** produce glucagon.
    o **Beta cells** produce insulin and amylin.
    o **Delta cells** produce somatostatin.
    o **Epsilon cells** produce **ghrelin**, which regulates hunger.
    o **PP cells** produce pancreatic polypeptide.

> **Helpful Hint**:
>
> **Exocrine glands** secrete substances into ducts so they can be transported to other parts of the body. The pancreas is both an endocrine and exocrine gland—it secretes hormones into the bloodstream and digestive juices into the pancreatic duct.

Practice Questions

6. Which type of pancreatic cells secrete insulin?

7. Which process does glucagon stimulate?

8. What affect does epinephrine have on blood glucose levels?

9. What is the normal level of glucose in the blood maintained by the process of glucose homeostasis?

10. Insulin lowers blood glucose levels by influencing which metabolic process?

Chapter 5 Answer Key

1. The pituitary gland secretes somatotropin.

2. Anabolic hormones stimulate cells to build large molecules by bonding smaller molecules together.

3. In a negative feedback loop, an external change prompts a response to return the body's internal environment to equilibrium.

4. During glycogenesis, glucose molecules bond together to make glycogen.

5. Glucose is the main sugar used during cellular respiration to produce molecules, such as ATP (adenosine triphosphate).

6. Insulin is secreted by the beta cells in the pancreatic islets.

7. Glucagon stimulates glycogenolysis, the breakdown of glycogen into glucose.

8. Epinephrine promotes the breakdown of glycogen and raises blood glucose levels.

9. Glucose homeostasis maintains blood glucose levels between 90 and 100 mg/dL.

10. Insulin stimulates glycogenesis, the storage of glucose molecules in the form of glycogen.

Chapter 6 – Person-Centered Planning

Individualized Education Plan and Goal Setting

Education plans should address all three learning domains: cognitive, affective, and psychomotor. For example, a patient who is learning about smoking cessation may need to be taught about the negative health impacts of smoking (cognitive domain), how to manage negative emotions related to quitting (affective domain), and how to correctly apply a nicotine patch (psychomotor domain).

The development of an **education plan** begins by assessing the patient's knowledge. A patient's knowledge can be formally assessed with a structured interview tool or written test, or less formally, during an initial discussion. The specialist should determine patients' education needs based on the following:

- medical condition

- previously acquired education

- willingness and ability to learn

Practice Question

1. Which of the learning domains should be addressed in an education plan?

Setting S.M.A.R.T. Goals

Once instruction is complete, the specialist and patient can work together to develop behavioral objectives, or measurable learning outcomes. Specialists should use the **S.M.A.R.T** acronym to develop behavioral objectives that are effective and likely to be met:

- **Specific:** The objective should be narrow and clearly defined.

- **Measurable:** The metrics for meeting the target should be defined.

- **Attainable:** The objective should be challenging but not unachievable.

- **Realistic:** The objective should be achievable within the context of the patient's needs and abilities.

- **Timeline:** A clear timeline for the objective should be defined.

For example, consider a patient recently diagnosed with type 2 diabetes who currently does not do any physical activity. After instruction on the definition and importance of physical activity, it is time for the patient to set a goal. The patient states, "My goal is to walk

> **Helpful Hint**:
>
> Patients are more likely to meet goals they have set themselves than goals that are set for them.

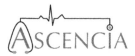

more." The specialist can then work with the patient to align this goal with the S.M.A.R.T model. An example of the resulting goal might be: "The patient will walk for at least thirty minutes three days a week. The specialist will follow up in four weeks to see if the patient is meeting the goal."

Practice Question

2. What are the elements of a S.M.A.R.T goal?

Achievement and Progress toward Goals

Follow-up after patient education is key to the continued success of a DSMES program. Specialists should follow ADCES guidelines for follow-up timelines. Typically, follow-ups should be conducted two to four weeks after the first session, then every three to six months afterwards.

To assess the success of the education program, the specialist should track **outcomes**—measurable results of education. Outcomes should be tracked over the immediate, intermediate, and long term.

Immediate outcomes include the acquisition of knowledge and skills. These learning outcomes can be measured immediately after instruction. The most common assessment tool is the **teach-back**, during which patients state what they have learned in their own words. Patients may also do **return demonstrations**, in which they demonstrate skills they have learned. **Oral** or **written tests** may be used to measure patient understanding, but many patients find these intimidating.

> **Helpful Hint**
>
> The ADCES provides tools on its website to help specialists measure outcomes related to each ADCES7 Self-Care Behavior.

Changes in behavior are **intermediate outcomes**. These outcomes are measured over a longer period of time and are compared to a baseline set during the initial assessment. **Post-intermediate outcomes** are clinical measures of health, such as BP or A1C. Improvements in these outcomes lead to long-term improvements in health and quality of life.

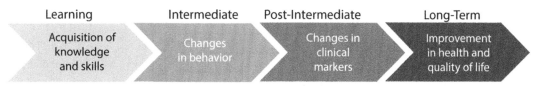

Figure 6.1. Learning Outcomes Continuum

Practice Questions

3. What are intermediate outcomes?

4. What do immediate outcomes measure?

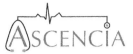

Nutrition Principles and Guidelines

Nutrition Recommendations

Nutrients are substances in food that are necessary for the growth, function, and maintenance of the human body. The energy derived from food is measured in **calories** (usually given in kilocalories [kcal]). Calories in food come mostly from **macronutrients** (also known as energy nutrients), which are needed in large quantities to sustain the body. There are three macronutrients:

- carbohydrates (4 kcal/g)

- fats (9 kcal/g)

- proteins (4 kcal/g)

> **Helpful Hint**:
>
> While alcohol yields 7 kcal/g, it is not a nutrient.

Micronutrients are vitamins (water- and fat-soluble) and minerals necessary for bodily processes. Important micronutrients include iron, calcium, vitamin A, vitamin D, iodine, folate, and zinc.

The amount and types of carbohydrates in packaged food can be found on the food's **nutrition facts label**. The FDA requires food manufacturers to include total carbohydrates, dietary fiber, total sugars, added sugars, and serving size on the nutrition label.

Nutrition Facts

8 servings per container

Serving size	2/3 cup (55g)

Amount per serving

Calories	230

	% Daily Value*
Total Fat 8g	10%
Saturated Fat 1g	5%
Trans Fat 0g	
Cholesterol 0mg	0%
Sodium 160mg	7%
Total Carbohydrate 37g	13%
Dietary Fiber 4g	14%
Total Sugars 12g	
Includes 10g Added Sugars	20%
Protein 3g	
Vitamin D 2mcg	10%
Calcium 260mg	20%
Iron 8mg	45%
Potassium 249mg	6%

*The % Daily Value (DV) tells you how much a nutrient in a serving of food contributes to a daily diet. 2,000 calories a day is used for general nutrition advice.

Figure 6.2. Nutrition Facts Label

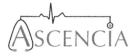

People with diabetes should also pay close attention to the list of ingredients in packaged foods, which is given in order of dominance of each ingredient. To help minimize sugar intake, patients should try to avoid foods that have added sugars (including syrups, honey, and fruit juice) listed in the first five ingredients.

Carbohydrates

Carbohydrates (sugars or saccharides) provide fuel for bodily processes. The consumption of carbohydrates raises blood glucose levels, so people with diabetes (PWD) must learn how to manage their carbohydrate intake to meet their blood glucose targets. Carbohydrates are generally broken up into three groups: sugars, starches, and fiber. Simple sugars are small molecules that can be quickly digested and used for energy:

- **Glucose** is the main source of energy for cellular processes.

- **Fructose** is a simple sugar that is converted to usable sources of energy (mainly glucose and glycogen) in the liver.

- **Sucrose** (white sugar) is a glucose and fructose molecule bonded together that is broken down into glucose in the body.

- **Lactose** is a glucose and a galactose molecule bonded together. It is found in milk and dairy products.

Plants store energy as **starch**, a polysaccharide composed of many glucose molecules bonded together. The body can digest starch, breaking it down into glucose. Common dietary sources of starch include cereal grains, root vegetables, and some beans, such as lentils and chickpeas.

Generally, a healthy dietary pattern will include nutrient-rich sources of carbohydrates that are also high in fiber, such as whole grains, fruits, and starchy vegetables. Non-starchy vegetables, which are low in carbohydrates (such as broccoli or okra), should also be included because they are nutrient-dense.

Carbohydrates from refined grains (as opposed to whole grains) should account for only a small amount of daily carbohydrate intake. **Refined grains** have had most of the fiber, micronutrients, and protein stripped away. Refined grains will cause a faster rise in blood glucose because the sugars are digested more quickly. White rice and white flour are both examples of refined grains.

Carbohydrate counting is a way for PWD to track the amount of carbohydrates they have consumed. It is especially important for people taking insulin since insulin doses should be matched to carbohydrate intake.

A serving of carbohydrates is 15 grams. The amount of a specific food that contains 15 grams of carbohydrates will vary based on the density of carbohydrates in that food. The following are examples of serving sizes with 15 grams of carbohydrates:

- $\frac{1}{3}$ cup pasta

- $\frac{1}{3}$ cup rice

- 3 cups popcorn (popped)

- 1 cup dairy milk

> **Helpful Hint**:
>
> Carbohydrate counting can be confusing, especially for patients with poor literacy or numeracy skills. The care plan should be customized for each patient to include the appropriate education and support with the skills needed to integrate carb counting into daily life.

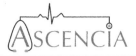

- 1 ounce whole-wheat or white sliced bread

- $\frac{1}{3}$ cup pinto beans

- $\frac{1}{2}$ banana

The number of carbohydrates suggested in a meal or day is individualized to meet patient preferences and glucose control. For example, a patient's care plan may suggest consuming fewer than 50 grams of carbohydrates in a meal. The patient would then count the carbohydrates in each food to stay within the 50 grams.

The **glycemic index** is a system designed to help PWD more easily track their carbohydrate intake. Research is mixed concerning its usefulness; some studies have shown it to help with blood glucose management while others have shown no positive impact.

In the glycemic index, carbohydrate foods are ranked from 0 to 100 by how quickly blood glucose rises after eating that food. The higher the index, the quicker a food is digested

> **Helpful Hint**:
>
> The freedom to choose from all carbohydrate sources can encourage patients to eat a variety of foods in varying amounts.

and the sugar absorbed into the bloodstream, leading to a rise in blood glucose. Pure glucose has a glycemic index of 100, while food with little sugar, such as nuts, have a glycemic index close to zero.

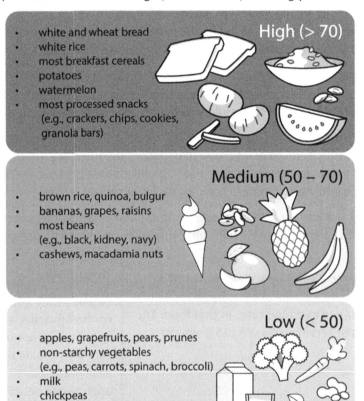

High (> 70)
- white and wheat bread
- white rice
- most breakfast cereals
- potatoes
- watermelon
- most processed snacks
  (e.g., crackers, chips, cookies, granola bars)

Medium (50 – 70)
- brown rice, quinoa, bulgur
- bananas, grapes, raisins
- most beans
  (e.g., black, kidney, navy)
- cashews, macadamia nuts

Low (< 50)
- apples, grapefruits, pears, prunes
- non-starchy vegetables
  (e.g., peas, carrots, spinach, broccoli)
- milk
- chickpeas
- peanuts, almonds, pecans, walnuts

Figure 6.3. The Glycemic Index

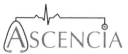

Because the glycemic index does not account for the amount of carbohydrates consumed, it does not accurately predict how a person's blood sugar will respond to a meal. More informative is the **glycemic load**, which is found by multiplying the grams of carbohydrates in a serving of food by the food's glycemic index, then dividing by 100. For example, the glycemic index of brown rice is 50, while its glycemic load is 10:

$$\text{Serving size:} \frac{1}{2} \text{ cup } = \text{ 20 grams of carbohydrates}$$

$$50 \times 20 = 1000 \div 100 = \mathbf{10}$$

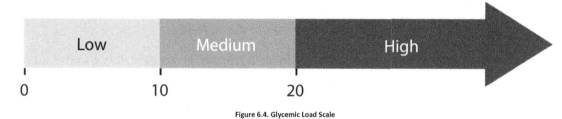

Figure 6.4. Glycemic Load Scale

Fiber

Dietary **fiber** consists of plant starches that cannot be digested. Consumption of fiber slows digestion, resulting in a slower rise in blood glucose following a meal. Fiber also feeds bacteria in the gut and provides bulk to stools. Fiber can be **soluble** (dissolvable in water) or **insoluble** (not dissolvable in water).

US Department of Health and Human Services Dietary Guidelines suggest that everyone, including people with diabetes (PWD), should get at least 14 grams of fiber per 1,000 kcal consumed. Good sources of fiber include whole grains, beans, nuts, and fruits and vegetables with their skin.

Fats

Fats (lipids) are used to store energy in the body. The primary lipid molecule found in the human body is **triglyceride**—three fatty acids bonded to one molecule of glycerol. Triglycerides can be saturated or unsaturated, with most foods containing a mix of the two.

Saturated fats have a high melting point and are usually solid at room temperature. Examples of foods high in saturated fats include whole milk, beef, and tropical oils like palm and coconut. Consuming these fats raises cholesterol levels and cardiovascular disease (CVD) risk, so most health guidelines suggest a dietary pattern low in saturated fats.

Unsaturated fats have a lower melting point and are typically liquid at room temperature. The majority of fats found in poultry, pork, fish, seafood, and most plants are unsaturated. Consumption of these fats is correlated with improved cardiovascular health. Unsaturated fats are further broken down into mono- and polyunsaturated based on their chemical structures:

> **Helpful Hint:**
>
> **Omega-3 fatty acids** are a type of polyunsaturated fatty acid found in fatty fish and some seeds, including flax and chia. Some evidence links consumption of omega-3 fatty acids to lowered risk of diabetes and CVD, although the relationship is still unclear.

- **Monounsaturated fats** are found in olive, canola, and sunflower oils; avocados; and many nuts.

- **Polyunsaturated fats** are found in sunflower and soybean oils, seeds, and fatty fish.

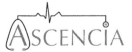

Trans fatty acids are created during the process of turning a liquid fat into a solid (e.g., turning vegetable oil into margarine). Consumption of trans fats lowers high-density lipoprotein (HDL) cholesterol, raises low-density lipoprotein (LDL) cholesterol, and is linked to an increased risk for CVD. Patients with diabetes should be encouraged to limit their intake of trans fats.

Cholesterol is another type of fat molecule that performs essential functions in the human body, including cell membrane support and the synthesis of hormones. As cholesterol travels through the blood it can adhere to blood vessels, leading to atherosclerosis. Most dietary guidelines recommend reducing the consumption of cholesterol to reduce the risk of CVD. Foods high in cholesterol include red meat, full-fat dairy products, and cooking oils.

Proteins

Protein is a nutrient that acts as the building block for cells, tissues, and organs. It is also the substrate used in the synthesis of hormones like insulin and glucagon. Proteins are macromolecules built from chains of **amino acids**. The human body builds proteins from twenty different amino acids. The body can manufacture eleven of these amino acids on its own; the other nine are **essential amino acids** that must be consumed. Protein can be consumed from both animal and plant sources:

- Animal sources of protein include meat, eggs, and dairy products.

- Plant products that are high in protein include soy products such as tempeh, tofu, soy milk, and edamame. Nuts, seeds, nutritional yeast, beans, peas, lentils, and whole grains also provide some protein.

> **Helpful Hint:**
>
> **Lean proteins** are sources of protein that are low in saturated fat and cholesterol. Sources of lean protein include poultry, pork, fish, and soy products.

The recommended dietary allowance (RDA) of protein for healthy adults is 0.8 grams per kilogram of body weight per day. Humans will need more in times of growth (i.e., pregnancy and childhood); trauma; illness; and wound healing.

Practice Questions

5. Where do most calories in food come from?

6. What is removed from the grain during the refining process?

7. What type of sugar is found in high amounts in dairy products?

8. What are the three types of carbohydrates?

9. What amount of cooked pasta contains approximately 15 grams of carbohydrates?

10. What is the recommended daily intake of fiber?

11. Rank the following foods in order from highest to lowest glycemic index: lentils, potatoes, eggplant, bananas.

12. What is the glycemic load for a $\frac{1}{2}$-cup serving of dried apricots? (Dried apricots contain 40 grams of carbohydrates per $\frac{1}{2}$ cup and have a glycemic index of 30.)

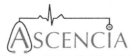

13. Which types of fats have been shown to increase LDL cholesterol levels and increase the risk for cardiovascular disease?

14. Which type of fat is most common in vegetables and fish?

15. Which types of food have high amounts of cholesterol?

16. What are essential amino acids?

17. What is the RDA of protein for healthy adults?

Food and Medication Integration

Managing morning hyperglycemia is challenging; it requires a careful balance of food and antidiabetic agents to avoid an overnight spike in BG. Management starts with data. Patients should use a BGM or measure BG at bedtime, at 2:00 a.m., and after waking up. The patient and specialist can use this data to test modifications to food or the scheduling and dosing of antidiabetic agents. The following general guidelines describe possible modifications, but changes will be specific to each patient:

- If BG is normal at bedtime and slowly rises, the patient may require a higher basal insulin dose.

- Patients with dawn phenomenon (BG normal at bedtime and high in the very early hours of the morning) may require an insulin pump. Simply increasing basal insulin may lead to overnight hypoglycemia.

- If BG is high at bedtime, patients may need to adjust their evening meals or snacks or increase insulin with their evening meals. Patients may also try light exercise after their evening meals to reduce BG levels.

Practice Question

18. What steps can patients take to help manage hyperglycemia at bedtime?

Special Considerations

Eating Disorders

Eating disorders are serious conditions marked by maladaptive dietary patterns that have negative impacts on health, emotions, and functioning. Some of the most common eating disorders include anorexia nervosa, bulimia nervosa, and binge-eating disorder. PWD may also develop eating disorders related to insulin use.

Anorexia nervosa is an eating disorder marked by an intense fear of gaining weight and a distorted body image. People with anorexia will control their weight by restricting their calorie intake through extreme dieting or by purging their calories through exercise, vomiting, and/or laxatives.

Helpful Hint:

While patients with anorexia are often underweight, specialists should recognize that overweight patients may also have anorexia, which is equally liable to impact their health and quality of life.

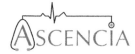

The long-term health effects of anorexia are very dangerous (e.g., organ failure) and sometimes fatal.

Bulimia nervosa is a life-threatening eating disorder marked by cycles of bingeing (excessive overeating) and purging. Binge eating is often done in short bursts, followed by purging through exercise, vomiting, and/or the use of laxatives or other drugs. People with bulimia are typically not underweight.

Binge-eating disorder is an eating disorder marked by periods of rapid excessive eating, often followed by feelings of intense shame, guilt, or disgust. Unlike people with bulimia, those with binge-eating disorder do not attempt to purge afterwards. The feelings of shame surrounding their eating can lead people to conduct binge sessions in private, where they will eat large amounts of food very quickly, past the point of discomfort.

Eating disorder–diabetes mellitus type 1 (ED-DMT1), also called **diabulimia**, is an eating disorder in which patients with type 1 diabetes restrict insulin use in order to lose weight. It is a serious condition that can lead to episodes of acute hyperglycemia and possibly diabetic ketoacidosis. The term *diabulimia* was created by the media and is not listed in the *Diagnostic and Statistical Manual of Mental Disorders* (fifth edition); however, it is sometimes classified as a purging behavior.

The following elements of diabetes care place patients at high risk for eating disorders:

- Diabetes is often managed through careful dietary patterns and tracking macronutrient intake. This type of food tracking can be a gateway to disordered eating.

- The high levels of stress experienced by people who self-manage their diabetes can lead to disordered eating habits.

- Patients who are overweight, particularly those with type 2 diabetes, are encouraged by medical providers to lose weight in order to prevent serious complications.

Eating disorders can be extremely dangerous for PWD because these disorders make it difficult to maintain glycemic control. PWD who also have eating disorders are at a higher risk of both acute and chronic complications and are more likely to experience chronic complications earlier in life.

Specialists should screen patients for eating disorders using a tool like the **Diabetes Eating Problem Survey—Revised (DEPS-R)**. Patients with symptoms of eating disorders should be referred for mental health care.

Practice Questions

19. What are the differences between bulimia nervosa and anorexia nervosa?

20. Explain the symptoms of binge-eating disorder.

Food Allergies and Failure to Thrive (FTT)

People with diabetes who suffer from autoimmune conditions, such as celiac disease must focus on gluten-free foods and make adjustments to avoid starchier foods, which can raise their blood sugar levels. PWD should focus on natural—not processed—gluten-free foods and select low-starch vegetables, lean meats, dairy, and fruits. Consultation with a registered dietitian nutritionist (RDN) is recommended.

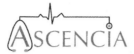

Patients with diabetes who experience food allergies may lack the nutritional awareness that is needed to improve their overall health and treat their conditions appropriately. Consequently, an individual with diabetes can develop a condition called **failure to thrive (FTT)**, which is caused by several factors that can lead to the following symptoms:

- weight loss

- increased fatigue

- inactivity

- depression

- memory loss

- decreased quality of life.

A diagnosis of adult failure to thrive typically begins with a doctor performing a physical exam, assessing chronic health problems, medication intake, and the patient's eating habits. Specifically, the physician can ask about the patient's change in daily activities. Medical problems such as diabetes, lack of food, and family issues related to poverty or neglect are contributors to FTT.

Diabetes can also interfere with the growth of pediatric patients, making them more susceptible to FTT. FTT is common and dangerous during the first three years of a child's active growth period. If the child is not growing in height and weight continuously, it can be a sign that the child is not eating enough food.

In addition to monitoring common FTT symptoms, physicians will also consult growth charts for specific age groups. The CDC provides several growth charts to monitor a patient's weight with respect to that person's age. For example, a 2-year-old child who initially weighs 15 kg (≈33 lb..) is projected to weigh 95 kg (≈210 lb.), on average, by the age of 20.

Practice Question

21. Which factors cause FTT?

Lifestyle Management

Specialists must help PWD understand how managing certain aspects of their lifestyle can support successful diabetes management.

Sleep and Stress

Sleep disturbance can be a critical challenge for proper type I or II diabetes self-management and care. For patients with type 2 diabetes, poor sleep is associated with poor diabetes self-care behaviors, which include exercise; diet (e.g., emotional eating); risk-reduction behaviors; and medication consumption.

Less healthy diets are generally associated with poor sleep quality and can occur when people with diabetes deviate from suggested meal plans. Adults with type 2 diabetes who experience insomnia will awaken more at night and will be tired during the day; consequently, diabetes self-care worsens. Adolescents with type 1 diabetes who have poor sleep quality tend to monitor blood glucose less frequently. Adolescents who oversleep are also less likely to monitor their blood glucose. Excess daytime sleepiness, as seen with patients who have had a longstanding diagnosis of type 2 diabetes, has

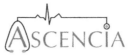

been linked to sedentary activity. Generally, seven hours of sleep per night is recommended. Improving circadian health can be done through time-restricted feeding, the use of melatonin, increasing physical activity/exercise, good sleep hygiene, and limited light exposure.

Stress can induce the release of several types of hormones, which can activate energy in the body to enable a fight-or-flight response. People with diabetes who have little or no insulin production and who experience emotional and/or environmental stress create stress hormones that increase their blood sugar levels. Consequently, glucose management and the body's inability to regulate the hormones will be difficult. Some studies have even linked a positive relationship between anxiety and the average blood sugar level (HbA1c) in adolescents with type 1 diabetes. In some cases, adolescents and adults with type 1 diabetes have reported raised blood sugar levels that have been associated with stressors such as video games, math problems, finances, job loss, and trauma. Each individual will perceive stress in various ways. The American Diabetes Association has listed several strategies to ease the stress of diabetes management. These strategies include challenging panicky thoughts, taking action, controlling breathing, having a mantra, having a happy place, exercising, meditating, expressing gratitude, making quality life choices, and taking warm baths.

Practice Questions

22. What are some ways to improve circadian health?

23. How does the fight-or-flight response affect blood sugar levels in people with diabetes?

Physical Activity

Development of an exercise program should start with an assessment of the patient's baseline exercise tolerance. To decrease the risk of injury, start low and slow: begin with low-intensity activities for a short time and gradually increase the intensity and time as tolerated by the patient.

The exercise program should also incorporate the activity preferences of the patient. Some patients may prefer structured exercise, such as aerobics classes, running, or biking; others may stay active through walking, cleaning, or gardening.

People with diabetes should spread the movements out over at least three days and not go more than two days without activity. The activity should last a minimum of ten minutes. Patients with diabetes should also be encouraged to get up from sitting every thirty minutes.

When developing a patient's management plan, specialists should assess barriers to activity. Lack of time, no place to exercise, and family commitments are frequent barriers listed by patients. Some patients may also have medical conditions that affect the amount and type of physical activity they can do. The specialist should work with patients to find activities that meet their needs.

> **Helpful Hint**:
>
> Specialists should note new complaints of exercise intolerance, which may be a sign of coronary artery disease or autonomic neuropathy.

Physical Activity: Benefits, Challenges, and Safety

Young adults with type 1 diabetes are generally less fit than individuals without diabetes; this can often be attributed to several comorbidities. For example, young patients with type 1 diabetes can have abnormalities in autonomic nerve functions and cardiac muscle in addition to reduced skeletal muscle size and power.

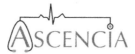

Since exercise requires more energy, the body will require more glucose, which can result in the onset of hypoglycemia. **Exercise-induced hypoglycemia (EIH)** is a condition where there is not enough glucose in the body to meet its energy requirements. Physicians define hypoglycemia as blood glucose below 70 milligrams per deciliter (mg/dl), but symptoms will result when the level drops below 55 mg/dL. Symptoms of EIH include fainting, dizziness, weakness, and anxiety. Individuals who take insulin or diabetes medication, do not consume enough carbohydrates, and drink alcohol without food are more likely to experience EIH.

People with diabetes who take medication when fasting can become hypoglycemic. The American Diabetes Association (ADA) suggests that PWD measure their blood glucose levels *before* exercising: if the glucose level is under 100 mg/dl, 15 – 20 grams of carbohydrates should be consumed to increase the level to at least 100 gm/dl. After 15 minutes of exercise, the glucose level should be checked again; consumption of carbohydrates is needed if the glucose levels are below the recommended amount.

Due to diabetes-related comorbidities and the susceptibility to EIH when exercising, PWD must eat regularly throughout the day and give the body enough time to adapt to new exercise routines. Studies have shown that anaerobic exercise, such as high-intensity training, was found to reduce hypoglycemia risks in young people with type 1 diabetes.

After exercise, PWD must consume carbohydrates to restore muscle and liver glycogen stores in order to avoid the onset of hypoglycemia. Individuals are advised to take snacks containing carbohydrates equal to about 1 gram per kilogram of body weight and proteins equal to about 0.3 grams per kilogram of body weight. The snacks should be taken with a third of the patient's insulin-to-carbohydrate ratio.

Practice Question

24. What are some common barriers to activity faced by patients with diabetes?

Self-Monitoring and Emergency Preparedness

Self-monitoring of blood glucose, specifically HbA1c measurements, for people with type 1 and 2 diabetes is important for maintaining blood glucose levels in order to reduce the risk of complications. Effective health care monitoring involves a partnership with the PWD and the specialist. Studies have resulted in simple and safe algorithms for adding and adjusting mealtime insulin. When self-monitoring is done correctly, glucose monitoring helps PWD assess their responses to therapy and achieve their target goals. Common sites for measurements include the finger, thumb, thigh, and forearm; measurements are recommended before each meal and before bedtime.

Glucose monitoring should be done up to 10 times a day during increased activity, illness, or post-surgery, and especially before driving. For people with type 1 diabetes who take several doses of insulin daily, carbohydrate counting combined with insulin dose adjustment is effective in lowering glycated hemoglobin (HbA1c), which improves quality of life and hypoglycemic episodes. Referral to structured educational food programs is recommended to ensure that carbohydrate counting and dietary advice are optimal. For PWD who are pregnant, maintaining an HBA1c level around 48 mmol/mol (6.5%) can reduce congenital malformations but can also increase the chances of hypoglycemia. For pediatric patients with type 1 and 2 diabetes, blood glucose levels must be monitored as they grow, and meal plans must be evaluated.

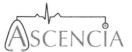

Hyperosmolar hyperglycemic syndrome and diabetic ketoacidosis are life-threatening emergencies. People with diabetes must be educated about the risks and strategies to prevent these conditions. Hyperglycemic emergencies, which can affect most patients with type 2 diabetes, are commonly caused by insulin omissions and errors as well as infection. **Bolus calculators** are commonly used tools to determine how much fast-acting insulin a patient needs before a meal. Friends and family members should be involved and educated about hyperglycemia, the sick day rule, and its management. In addition to having medical wristbands, close relatives should have medical supplies, insulin storage, and diabetes emergency kits. Relatives should also know how to administer glucagon treatment if the patient with diabetes becomes unconscious.

Children with diabetes should have a school health plan in place that includes contact information for family members as well as the child's diabetes care provider or specialist. The health plan should contain routine information on diabetes management, such as insulin administration/dosing, snack times, and blood glucose monitoring. Emergency plans for the management of hyper- or hypoglycemia should be included as well as scenarios where there can be issues with insulin pumps or pump failures.

Practice Question

25. People with diabetes are encouraged to monitor their blood glucose levels to adjust for food intake and pharmacological therapy in order to reach their target goals. What are the recommended times of day to perform self-monitoring?

26. What are the most common causes of hyperglycemic emergencies?

School

School environments can present a challenge for children who need to manage their diabetes. Older children may be able to check their own BG levels and administer insulin, but younger children will require care from trained school staff.

All students with diabetes should have a **diabetes medical management plan (DMMP)** that has been completed by the child's parents and medical provider. The DMMP is implemented by the school nurse or other health professional who can ensure that the child's individual care needs are met. The DMMP includes the following information:

- detailed plan for glucose monitoring
- medication types and dosages
- directions for the management of meals, snacks, and exercise
- plan for treating hypoglycemia, hyperglycemia, and other emergencies
- details about the child's self-management skills

The Americans with Disabilities Act requires schools to provide accommodations to students with diabetes. Schools must provide trained staff who can monitor BG and administer medications, including during field trips. They must also allow students to self-manage their

> **Helpful Hint**:
>
> A 504 plan, which is developed to provide accommodations to students with disabilities, is different from an **individualized education plan (IEP)**. IEPs focus more on learning goals and specialized instruction for the student; these are not included in a 504 plan.

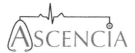

diabetes to the extent that they and their families deem them capable and willing. Schools cannot do the following:

- prevent students from going on field trips because of a lack of available staff

- require students to transfer schools

- require family members to come to school to provide care

Students with diabetes may have a **504 plan**. Section 504 is part of the Rehabilitation Act of 1973, which requires all students to have access to free appropriate public education. A 504 plan details the child's care plan and also lists accommodations the school will provide the student (e.g., trained personnel, meal/beverage breaks).

Practice Question

27. What document should be filled out by the student's medical provider and parents to inform the school about the student's diabetes care needs?

Medication Management and Insulin

ADA/European Association for the Study of Diabetes (EASD) Guidelines

Both the American Diabetes Association (ADA) and the European Association for the Study of Diabetes (EASD) have created consensus statements on the management of hyperglycemia for patients with type 2 diabetes. The main consensus recommendations state that providers/health care systems should prioritize delivering patient-centered care.

Patients with type 2 diabetes should be offered access to specific self-management education and support programs (e.g., DSMES). The ADA and EASD recommend a stepwise approach to glycemic control that begins with metformin with gradual intensification to dual/triple therapy of glucose-lowering medications. The ADA/EASD guidelines for glycemic targets are more user-friendly for practitioners due to the stepwise intensification regimens. Individualized glycemic targets for people with diabetes will depend on life expectancy, comorbidity, and resources. In contrast, the AACE/ACE guidelines are stricter and more commonly followed by specialists.

Practice Question

28. What is the prevailing consensus from both the ADA and the EASD concerning the management of hyperglycemia for patients with type 2 diabetes?

Medications and Medication Selections

Patients with type 2 diabetes who have insufficient endogenous insulin can administer antidiabetic agents and exogenous insulin to better cope with insulin resistance. Metformin is the main drug used for people with Type 2 diabetes. Dipeptidyl peptidase-4 inhibitors and glucagon-like peptide-1 receptor antagonists combined with metformin and sulfonylurea derivative oral agents can significantly improve

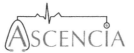

glycemic levels in people with type 1 diabetes as well as people with type 2 diabetes. Some people with diabetes have allergies to medication such as metformin, and others with kidney disease must seek other therapies. Both the ADA and EASD recommend second-line therapies after the use of metformin; the second-line therapy chosen is based on kidney and cardiovascular comorbidities, hypoglycemia, weight gain, and cost. SGLT-2 inhibitors are alternatives that can lower blood pressure and reduce cardiovascular issues while also lowering blood glucose.

The glycemic efficacy of SGLT-2 inhibitors is modest and limits renal function decline. The benefits of these inhibitors are that there is no increased risk of hypoglycemia, and there is modest blood pressure lowering and weight loss. In the US and Europe, these inhibitors have been approved by regulatory authorities, such as the FDA, and are sold under the following medication names:

- ertugliflozin

- empagliflozin

- canagliflozin

- dapagliflozin

Practice Question

29. What is an alternative to metformin that can lower blood pressure and blood glucose as well as reduce cardiovascular issues?

Immunizations

Diabetes makes people more susceptible to infection through a number of different mechanisms:

- The body's natural immunological response is impaired by high BG levels, making it harder to fight off infections.

- Peripheral neuropathy allows skin lesions to be overlooked or disregarded until an infection develops.

- Autonomic neuropathy in the digestive tract and urinary system delays emptying, allowing infections to take hold there.

- Frequent testing, medical procedures, and hospitalization related to diabetes care increase the risk of infection.

- Vascular damage restricts blood supply to specific areas, which slows healing.

As with other complications, tight management of BG and BP levels can help reduce the chances of serious illnesses. People with diabetes should take care to limit opportunities for infection and treat infections early. This management may include foot and skin checks, prompt treatment of autonomic neuropathy, and **vaccinations**. According to the ADA, adults with diabetes should routinely receive the following vaccinations:

- annual influenza vaccine

- pneumococcal polysaccharide vaccine for all PWD ages 2 and older; a one-time revaccination for individuals older than 64 who were previously immunized more than 5 years ago and were under age 65 at the time; repeat vaccination indicated for nephritic syndrome, chronic renal disease, and other immunocompromised states, such as after transplantation

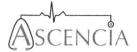

- hepatitis B vaccination for unvaccinated adults

- tetanus and diphtheria vaccinations every 10 years

- herpes zoster, recombinant vaccine, for PWD ages 50 and over

- SARS-CoV-2 vaccination, with booster vaccination per latest Centers for Disease Control and Prevention guidelines

For adults with diabetes, additional vaccinations against hepatitis A, varicella, and meningitis may be advised depending on the patient's medical history.

Practice Questions

30. How frequently should someone with T1D receive the influenza vaccine?

31. How can autonomic neuropathy lead to increased risk of infection?

Insulin and Its Pharmacology

Insulin is released at a steady rate, called the **basal rate**, which is estimated to be 0.5 – 1 unit/hour. Insulin is also released after food is eaten. The increase in BG that occurs after eating stimulates the pancreas to release insulin in a biphasic release pattern with two waves:

1. Within minutes of a meal, the pancreas secretes a bolus, or fast release of insulin, to facilitate a quick uptake of glucose into the cells.

2. The second wave of insulin is released gradually to manage the additional glucose load that occurs as the meal digests over time.

To achieve glycemic targets in patients with diabetes, insulin can be injected to mimic endogenous (produced within a system) patterns. Basal insulin is used to control BG levels between meals. Bolus insulin (also called mealtime insulin) is used to manage the additional glucose load associated with eating.

What differentiates basal and bolus insulin products is their respective pharmacokinetics, or how the insulin acts in the body. The three key parameters that define insulin's pharmacokinetic profile are onset, peak, and duration:

- **Onset** describes the moment when insulin begins to take effect in the body.

- The point at which insulin is exerting its maximum effect is called the **peak**.

- The **duration**, or **duration of action (DOA)**, is the length of time insulin remains at work in the body.

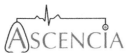

Basal insulin has a slower onset, no peak (i.e., flattened curve), and a longer DOA. In contrast, bolus insulin has a faster onset, an evident and sharp peak, and shorter DOA.

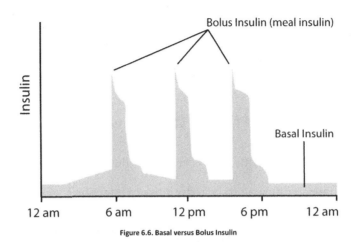

Figure 6.6. Basal versus Bolus Insulin

Insulin dosing is measured in units, or international units (IU). A unit of insulin is equivalent to 0.0347 mg of pure crystalline insulin.

Insulin products are provided in concentrations of units per milliliter. For example, an insulin pen may have a concentration of 100 units/mL ("U-100"), meaning that each milliliter contains 100 units. If the dose for a patient is 10 units, then the correct volume of the dose is 0.1 milliliter:

- $10 \text{ units } \times \frac{1 \text{ mL}}{100 \text{ units}} = 0.1 \text{ mL}$

If a U-100 pen has a total of 3 mL of fluid, then the number of units in the pen would be 300 units:

- $U - 100 = 100 \text{ units per } 1 \text{ mL}$

- $3 \text{ mL } \times \frac{100 \text{ units}}{1 \text{ mL}} = 300 \text{ units}$

Practice Questions

32. What is the difference in DOA for basal versus bolus insulin?

33. What term describes the point at which insulin is exerting its maximum effect?

34. A patient is taking Humalog (bolus insulin) 4 units subcutaneous (SQ) before dinner and Lantus (basal insulin) 20 units SQ at bedtime. Lantus and Humalog each come as a 3 mL pen with a concentration of 100 units/mL. How many milliliters of insulin is this patient injecting before dinner and at bedtime?

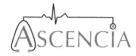

Types of Insulin

Human insulin is the term used to describe synthetic insulin that has the same amino acid sequence as endogenous insulin. Human insulin does not perform the same as endogenous insulin once injected; it has a delayed onset and more variable peak and DOA.

Insulin analogs are synthetic insulins with a modified amino acid sequence. They perform the same action as endogenous insulin but are modified to have varying onsets, peaks, and DOAs. These modifications are usually achieved by changing the way insulin interacts with zinc.

> **Helpful Hint**:
>
> Insulin is often referred to as the "key" that allows glucose to enter cells. Without insulin, cells can starve even as BG levels increase within the bloodstream.

Insulin bonds with zinc in the blood to form **hexamers**, which cannot bind to receptors. The hexamers must break down before the insulin can be used by cells. Insulin analogs interact with zinc in different ways to make insulin more quickly available (by preventing hexamer formation) or to make insulin's duration longer (by slowing the breakdown of hexamers).

Table 4.1. Pharmacokinetics of Insulin Injectables

Type	Insulin (Brand Names)	Onset (hrs)	Peak (hrs)	Duration of Action (hrs)	When to Inject
Rapid-acting	insulin lispro (Humalog) insulin aspart (Novolog) insulin glulisine (Apidra)	0.25 – 0.5	0.5 – 2.5	3 – 5	15 – 20 min before meals
Short-acting	regular insulin (Humulin R, Novolin R)	0.5 – 1	2 – 3	8	30 minutes before meals
Intermediate-acting	human insulin neutral protamine Hagedorn (NPH) (Humulin N, Novolin N)	1 – 2	4 – 10	10 – 16	single dose usually at bedtime or in 2 divided doses

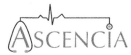
Table 4.1. Pharmacokinetics of Insulin Injectables					
Type	Insulin (Brand Names)	Onset (hrs)	Peak (hrs)	Duration of Action (hrs)	When to Inject
Long-acting	insulin glargine (**Lantus, Basaglar, Semglee, Toujeo**) insulin detemir* (**Levemir**)	1 – 9	none	up to 24	once daily at patient's convenience, usually either in the morning or evening** insulin detemir: once daily in the evening or in 2 divided doses daily
Ultra-long-acting	insulin degludec (**Tresiba**)	9	none	36 – 48	once daily at patient's convenience, usually either in the morning or evening
*DOA for insulin detemir is dose dependent and varies from 6 to 23 hours. At lower doses of 0.1 – 0.2 units per kilogram of body weight (units/kg), DOA ranges from 5.7 to 12.1 hours. At higher doses of ≥0.8 units/kg, the DOA is longer, between 22 and 23 hours.					
**Lantus U-100 can be dosed twice daily as its DOA can range from 10 to 24 hours.					

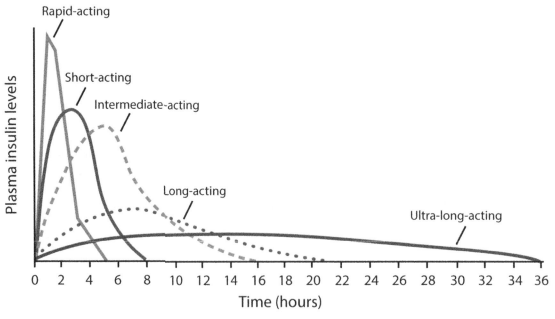

Figure 6.7. Pharmacokinetics of Insulin Products

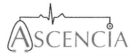

Fixed combinations of insulin contain basal and bolus components. Fixed insulin regimens can be considered in patients who require both basal and bolus insulin and who would benefit from a simpler injection regimen and lower cost. Premixed combinations include the following:

- NovoLog Mix 70/30 (70% insulin aspart protamine and 30% insulin aspart)

- Novolin 70/30 (70% insulin NPH and 30% regular insulin)

- Humulin 50/50 (50% insulin NPH and 50% regular insulin)

- Humulin 70/30 (70% insulin NPH and 30% regular insulin)

- Humalog Mix 75/25 (75% insulin lispro protamine and 25% insulin lispro)

- Humalog Mix 50/50 (50% insulin lispro protamine and 50% insulin lispro)

- Ryzodeg 70/30 (70% insulin degludec and 30% insulin aspart)

Afrezza, an **inhaled insulin**, is an ultra-rapid-acting insulin with an onset of around 12 minutes, peak of 35 – 50 minutes, and a DOA of 1.5 – 4.5 hours. Afrezza is taken at the beginning of the meal and has a boxed warning for acute bronchospasm. It should be avoided in patients with chronic lung disease, such as COPD and asthma. Coughing is a common side effect.

> **Helpful Hint**:
>
> Fixed combinations of insulin are generally avoided in patients with type 1 diabetes due to the need for frequent adjustments to mealtime insulin doses.

Practice Questions

35. What is the order—from fastest- to longest-acting—of the following: regular insulin, insulin NPH, Lantus, Novolog?

36. At what time of day should a patient take Afrezza?

37. What is the DOA for insulin glargine?

38. When should patients inject rapid-acting insulin, such as Humalog or Novolog?

39. What type of patient would MOST benefit from a fixed-dose insulin regimen?

Insulin Dosing

A patient with T1D will typically require a **total daily dose (TDD)** of insulin of 0.4 – 1.0 units/kg/day. For example, if a 70 kg patient needs to administer 0.5 units/kg/day, the total daily insulin dose is 35 units.

> **Helpful Hint**:
>
> Patients can find their personal insulin-to-carb ratio by closely tracking how many grams of carbohydrates they ate, how much insulin they took, and their BG levels before and after the meal.

Approximately 40% – 50% of the TDD is basal insulin administered to replace insulin overnight. The basal insulin dose is typically constant from day to day. The remaining balance of 50% – 60% of TDD is bolus insulin replacement for carbohydrate coverage and high blood sugar correction. The required dosage of bolus insulin will vary with diet and activity.

Patients should know their **insulin-to-carb ratio**, which is the amount (in grams) of carbohydrates covered by one unit of

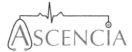

rapid-acting insulin. This number varies with each patient; typically, one unit of rapid-acting insulin will cover 12 – 15 grams of carbohydrates, but this value can be lower or much higher, depending on insulin sensitivity.

An **insulin correction factor** is the amount that one unit of rapid-acting insulin will lower a patient's BG level. For example, an insulin correction factor of 40 means that one unit of rapid-acting insulin will lower the patient's BG by 40 mg/dL. This number is specific to each patient. The insulin correction factor is used to bring down BG levels that are out of target range:

$$\text{target BG} = 120 \text{ mg/dL}$$

$$\text{current BG} = 200 \text{ mg/dL}$$

$$\text{insulin correction factor} = 40 \text{ mg/dL/unit}$$

$$\text{insulin dose} = (200 - 120) \div 40 = 2 \text{ units}$$

Patients may also use a **sliding scale** to correct for high BG. A sample is shown in Table 6.2. The scale may be adjusted for patients with higher or lower insulin sensitivities.

Table 6.2. Sample Sliding Scale for Correction Insulin	
Blood Glucose (mg/dL)	**Insulin Units**
<150	0
151 – 200	2
201 – 250	4
251 – 300	6
301 – 350	8
>350	10

The three case studies which follow provide examples of how the many types of insulin can be used to manage patients with different types of diabetes, blood glucose levels, and lifestyles.

Case 1: Basal Only

A 45-year-old woman who was diagnosed with T2D 5 years ago presents to her primary care physician for a follow-up. The patient is already optimized on a triple therapy with metformin, pioglitazone, and glipizide; however, she has not met her A1C target. Her average fasting blood glucose (FBG) is 195 and her A1C is 7.9%. She is initiated on Lantus 10 units SQ once daily.

Explanation: The patient has tried triple therapy and has still not met her A1C target. Per American Diabetes Association (ADA) guidelines, she should be started on either a basal insulin or bedtime Neutral Protamine Hagedorn (NPH) insulin. Lantus is a long-acting basal insulin analog that can be titrated by 2 units every 3 days to achieve the FBG target. In the future, the patient may benefit from mealtime insulin; however, she would need to be evaluated at her next follow-up and have pre- or postprandial readings.

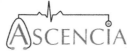

Case 2: Basal + Bolus

A 27-year-old man with T1D receives a TDD of 0.5 units of insulin per kg/day. He weighs 96 kg. His TDD is 50% bolus insulin and 50% basal. He uses 8 units before each meal.

Explanation: The patient uses a total of 48 units of insulin per day. TDD is calculated as follows:

- total daily dose (TDD) $= 96 \text{ kg} \times 0.5 \text{ units/kg/day} = 48 \text{ units per day}$

Fifty percent of the TDD is basal insulin. One-half of 48 units is 24 units of basal insulin per day.

Fifty percent of the TDD is bolus insulin. One-half of 48 units is 24 units of bolus insulin per day. His bolus insulin is divided evenly to be administered before meals.

- $24 \text{ units per day} \div 3 \text{ meals per day} = 8 \text{ units before each meal}$

Case 3: Fixed Regimen

A 62-year-old man has uncontrolled type 2 diabetes that was diagnosed 6 months ago. Past medical history includes heart failure. He takes metformin 500 mg orally once daily and cannot tolerate higher doses. He desires a cost-effective option. His A1C is 9.8%, average FBG is 187, and average postprandial glucose (PPG) is 234. The doctor initiates the patient on Humulin 70/30 10 units SQ twice daily and counsels the patient to increase the total daily insulin by 2 units every 3 days until BG targets are achieved.

Explanation: Additional therapy is needed, but the patient cannot tolerate higher metformin doses. Because of the patient's history of heart failure, pioglitazone should be avoided even though it is a cost-effective glucose-lowering therapy. Access to glucagon-like peptide-1 (GLP-1) and sodium-glucose cotransporter-2 (SGLT2) inhibitor therapy may be cost prohibitive. The patient needs both basal and mealtime control to meet BG targets. Of the insulin products available, a relatively cost-effective option is premixed Humulin 70/30 containing NPH and regular insulin.

Practice Questions

40. What is a typical insulin-to-carb ratio?

41. What percentage of the total daily insulin dose is usually basal insulin?

Insulin Delivery Systems and Injection Techniques

Insulin injection options for SQ delivery include a vial with syringe, pens, and pumps.

An **insulin vial with syringe** is the most frequently used method of delivery. It is less expensive than the pen or pump, and some syringes allow insulin mixing. Drawbacks of this method include difficulty in reading the marked increments and inconvenience when traveling.

Insulin from vials must be drawn into a syringe. Then, the patient (or person administering the insulin) pinches the skin and inserts the syringe at a 45-degree angle. Depending on adiposity and needle size, the injection may be also done at a 90-degree angle. The needle should be kept in place for about 5 seconds to ensure insulin delivery.

Insulin pens are prefilled and require fewer steps than the vial and syringe methods. They allow for more accurate dosing and are discreet to carry; however, insulin pens are more expensive, and not all

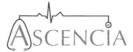

insulin types are available in pens. Insulins in pens cannot be mixed, though some pens come with premixed formulations.

In general, insulin pens are injected at a 90-degree angle using the dominant hand, with fingers wrapped around the pen and the thumb free to press the knob. The knob must be pressed down all the way. It is important to count 6 to 10 seconds before withdrawing the pen.

Both syringes and pens can be injected in multiple body parts. Insulin is absorbed fastest when injected in the abdomen. The next fastest-absorbing injection site is the back of the upper arm, followed by the thighs. The buttocks absorb insulin the slowest.

The rate of absorption of rapid- and long-acting insulin is similar in different body parts, so patients may choose to rotate injection sites. The rate of absorption of intermediate-acting and premixed insulin differs across body parts, so it is best for patients to inject these insulins into the same general body part, rotating to different specific sites.

Regardless of the insulin product, certain best practices of proper injection techniques should be observed. Patients should always do the following:

- wash their hands prior to injection

- rotate the injection site to avoid adverse events, such as lipohypertrophy

- not inject into areas that are tender, bruised, lumpy, numb, or firm

- not rub or apply heat to the injection site

Helpful Hint:

Injections need to be about 2 inches away from the navel or belly button to avoid sensitive and painful areas.

Insulin pumps mimic the function of the pancreas by supplying the delivery of SQ basal and bolus insulins. They provide convenient, precise, and simplified insulin dosing. Patients using pumps are at a lower risk of severe hypoglycemia. Drawbacks include the expense of the of the pumps and supplies, risk of infection, and inconvenience of the tubing.

Helpful Hint:

Manufacturers of insulin pens, such as Lantus SoloStar and Tresiba FlexTouch, provide instructional videos.

The traditional pump includes a device with a reservoir of insulin that is either placed in a pocket or strapped to the patient's clothes. A tube connects the device to a cannula or needle that is secured by a hypoallergenic adhesive. A

Chapter 6 – Person-Centered Planning

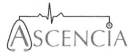

continuous glucose monitoring sensor is placed on the patient and transmits data to the pump itself or to another device, such as a smartphone.

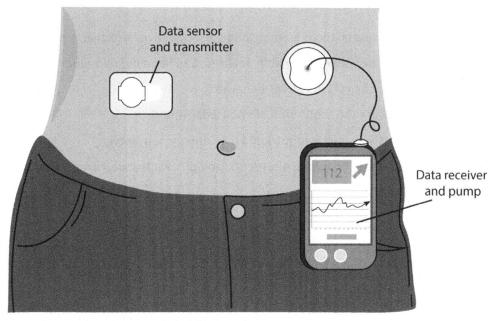

Figure 6.8. Typical Setup of a Traditional Pump with CGM

A **patch pump** is a tubeless pump that contains the insulin reservoir, batteries, and cannula that delivers SQ insulin. A remote device, called a personal diabetes manager, controls how much insulin is delivered.

> **Helpful Hint**:
>
> An insulin pump's infusion set and site of infusion should be changed every 2 – 3 days.

Practice Questions

42. How long should patients hold the needle in place after injecting insulin?

43. Which injection site absorbs insulin the fastest?

44. How often should patients change the infusion set and site if using a traditional pump?

Chapter 6 Answer Key

1. Education plans should address all three learning domains: cognitive, affective, and psychomotor.

2. A SMART goal is specific, measurable, attainable, realistic, and has a defined timeline.

3. Intermediate outcomes are changes in patient behaviors.

4. Immediate outcomes measure the acquisition of knowledge and skills.

5. Calories in food come mostly from **macronutrients** (i.e., energy nutrients).

6. Refined grains have most of the fiber, micronutrients, and protein stripped away.

7. Dairy products contain lactose.

8. The three types of carbohydrates are sugars, starches, and fiber.

9. A serving size of $\frac{1}{3}$ cup of cooked pasta contains approximately 15 grams of carbohydrates.

10. The recommended daily intake of fiber is 14 grams of fiber per 1,000 kcal consumed.

11. The foods ranked from highest to lowest glycemic index: potatoes, bananas, lentils, eggplant.

12. Calculate the glycemic load: glycemic index = 30 serving size = 1/2 cup = 40 grams of carbohydrates $30 \times 40 = 1200 \div 100 = 12$.

13. Saturated and trans fats raise low-density lipoprotein (LDL) cholesterol and cardiovascular disease (CVD) risk.

14. Vegetables and fish contain mostly unsaturated fats.

15. Foods high in cholesterol include red meat, full-fat dairy products, and cooking oils.

16. Essential amino acids are those which cannot be manufactured by the human body and must be consumed.

17. The recommended dietary allowance (RDA) of protein for healthy adults is 0.8 grams per kilogram of body weight per day.

18. Patients with hyperglycemia at bedtime can adjust their evening meals or snacks or increase insulin with their evening meal. They can also try light exercise after their evening meal to reduce blood glucose (BG) levels.

19. Patients with bulimia go through cycles of bingeing and purging, while those with anorexia do not binge.

20. Binge-eating disorder is characterized by periods of rapid excessive eating to the point of physical pain, followed by periods of intense shame and guilt.

21. Failure to thrive (FTT) is caused by weight loss, increased fatigue, inactivity, depression, memory loss, and decreased quality of life.

22. Circadian health can be improved through time-restricted feeding, using melatonin, increasing physical activity/exercise, having good sleep hygiene, and having limited light exposure.

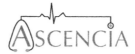

23. In people with diabetes, the fight-or-flight response causes them to create stress hormones that increase their blood sugar levels.

24. Patients may cite lack of time, no place to exercise, and family commitments as barriers to activity; they may also have medical conditions that limit their ability to exercise.

25. Ideally, PWD should measure their blood glucose levels at least four times a day: three times before each meal and before going to bed.

26. Hyperglycemic emergencies are most often caused by insulin omissions, errors, and infection.

27. A diabetes medical management plan (DMMP) is completed by the student's parents and medical provider every year.

28. The main consensus recommendations state that delivering patient-centered care should always be the priority.

29. SGLT-2 inhibitors are alternatives to metformin that can lower blood pressure and reduce cardiovascular issues while also lowering blood glucose.

30. A patient with type 1 diabetes (T1D) needs to get a flu shot annually.

31. Autonomic neuropathy in the digestive tract and urinary system delays emptying, allowing infections to take hold there.

32. Basal insulin has a longer duration of action (DOA) than bolus insulin.

33. The *peak* is the point at which insulin is exerting its maximum effect.

34. The patient is injecting 0.04 mL of Humalog and 0.2 mL of Lantus:

$$\text{Humalog: 4 units} \times \frac{1\text{ mL}}{100\text{ units}} = 0.04\text{ mL}$$

$$\text{Lantus: 20 units} \times \frac{1\text{ mL}}{100\text{ units}} = 0.2\text{ mL}$$

35. The correct order from fastest- to longest-acting is Novolog, regular insulin, insulin NPH, and Lantus.

36. Patients should take Afrezza at the start of their meals.

37. Insulin glargine has a duration of action (DOA) of up to 24 hours.

38. Patients should inject rapid-acting insulin, such as Humalog or Novolog, 15 to 20 minutes before their meals.

39. Fixed-dose insulin regimens can be considered in patients who require both basal and bolus therapy and who may benefit from lower costs and simpler injection regimens.

40. One unit of rapid-acting insulin covers 12 – 15 grams of carbohydrates (1:12 – 1:15).

41. Basal insulin typically accounts for 40% – 50% of the total daily dose (TDD) of insulin.

42. After injecting insulin with a pen, patients should hold the needle and count 6 – 10 seconds; when using a syringe, they should count about 5 seconds to ensure proper delivery.

43. The abdomen absorbs insulin the fastest.

44. The infusion set and site must be changed every 2 – 3 days with a traditional pump.

Chapter 7 – Monitoring, Interpretation, and Acute Complications

A1C and Glycemic Metrics

The benchmark metric for assessing long-term glycemic control is A1C, which represents the average blood glucose level over the previous 3 months. People with diabetes should have their A1C regularly checked:

- Patients with stable glycemic control should have their A1C tested at least twice a year.

- Patients with poor glycemic control, or those who have recently adjusted their management plans, should be tested at least 4 times a year.

The most common A1C goal is <7%. This target may be reduced if the patient responds well to treatment and is at low risk for hypoglycemia. Some patients may benefit from looser glycemic control with a target A1C of <8% if the harms of treatment outweigh the benefits.

Fructosamine is a rarely used glycation marker that shows glucose levels over the previous 2 – 3 weeks. Testing fructosamine levels may be helpful if a patient's red blood cells have a shortened life span, which can make A1C results unreliable; however, it is not a screening test for diabetes.

A monosaccharide that circulates in the blood is **1,5 anhydroglucitol (1,5-AG)**, which competes with glucose for kidney reabsorption. During hyperglycemia, 1,5-AG is excreted in the urine and its levels in the blood drop. The 1,5-AG level can show increases in blood sugar not detected in BG or A1C levels; if hyperglycemia has occurred within the past 2 weeks, there will be a decrease in the 1,5-AG level.

Practice Questions

1. What is the most common target A1C range for PWD?

2. What does a decrease in the level of 1,5-AG indicate?

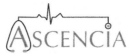

Blood Pressure

Blood pressure (BP) is the pressure exerted by blood on the inside of blood vessels. **Systolic blood pressure (SBP)** is the pressure that occurs while the heart is contracting. **Diastolic blood pressure (DBP)** occurs while the heart is relaxed.

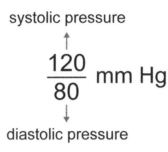

systolic pressure

$$\frac{120}{80} \text{ mm Hg}$$

diastolic pressure

Figure 7.1. Systolic and Diastolic Blood Pressures

Hypertension—high blood pressure—is linked to the development of CVD. In patients with diabetes, hypertension is also linked to worsening diabetic complications, including neuropathy, retinopathy, and nephropathy. The ADA recommends intervention for patients with elevated BP, with increasing levels of intervention for higher BP.

> **Helpful Hint**:
>
> Measurements of more than 140/90 mmHg at one office visit should be repeated on a separate day before diagnosing hypertension. Only one reading is needed for diagnosing high blood pressure if the level is ≥180/110 mmHg.

Table 7.1. Levels of Intervention for Hypertension

Blood Pressure Category	BP Range (mmHg)	Intervention
Normal	<120/80	none
Elevated/stage 1 hypertension	SBP: 120 – 139 DBP: <80	lifestyle modifications
Stage 2 hypertension	SBP: 140 – 159 DBP: >90	lifestyle modifications plus one BP drug
	SBP: 160 – 179 DBP: >90	lifestyle modifications plus two BP drugs
Hypertensive crisis	SBP: >180 DBP: >120 with signs and symptoms of organ failure	emergency intervention with oral or IV drugs to lower BP

Target ranges should be adapted to each individual patient. Generally, for patients with low risk of cardiovascular disease, the recommended BP target is under 140/90 mmHg. Patients with higher risk

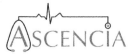

may benefit from a lower target of 130/80 mm Hg or lower. The ADA target for pregnant patients with preexisting hypertension is between 110/85 and 135/85 mmHg.

All patients with BP higher than 120/80 mmHg should be educated on lifestyle modifications, such as the following, that can help decrease BP:

- the DASH diet

- regular physical activity

- losing excess weight

- smoking cessation

- avoiding excessive alcohol consumption (men: more than two alcoholic beverages per day; women: more than one alcoholic beverage per day)

One medication is initiated if blood pressure levels are over 140/90 mmHg and lower than 160/100 mmHg. Two medications are used for treatment if levels are 160/90 mmHg or higher. For both categories, lifestyle interventions are included with medications .

The choice of medications is based on the patient's underlying conditions and tolerance for medications. Generally, PWD are prescribed an angiotensin-converting enzyme (ACE) inhibitor or angiotensin II receptor blocker as a first-line medication. Other drugs, including calcium channel blockers and diuretics, may be added to this regimen. These medications are discussed in detail in Table 7.2.

> **Helpful Hint**:
>
> All patients with diabetes and hypertension should monitor their blood pressure at home. The use of digital apps or websites can help patients effectively monitor and track their BP.

Table 7.2. Pharmacological Management of Blood Pressure		
Category of Drug	**Action**	**Adverse Reactions and Interactions**
ACE inhibitors lisinopril (Prinivil, Zestril) benazepril (Lotensin) enalapril (Epaned, Vasotec)	block the ACE to prevent vasoconstriction and relax blood vessels	BBW*: fetal toxicity ADR**: cough, hypotension, dizziness
Angiotensin II receptor blockers (A2RBs) losartan (Cozaar) valsartan (Diovan)	block angiotensin II receptor site; prevent vasoconstriction and relax blood vessels	BBW: fetal toxicity ADR: dizziness, headache, fatigue interactions: potassium supplements pregnancy: category D
Calcium channel blockers (CCBs) Amlodipine (Amvaz, Norvasc)	block movement of calcium in vascular muscles, relaxing blood vessels	ADR: headache, edema, tiredness, dizziness interactions: grapefruit (nifedipine)

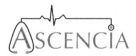

Category of Drug	Action	Adverse Reactions and Interactions
Diltiazem (Cardizem) Nifedipine (Procardia)		
Diuretics hydrochlorothiazide (Microzide) furosemide (Lasix) spironolactone (Aldactone, CaroSpir)	prevent reabsorption in kidneys, resulting in increased urination and fluid loss	BBW: fluid/electrolyte loss (furosemide), fetal toxicity (lisinopril) ADR: hypotension, weakness, dizziness, blurred vision due to fluid loss from increased urination interactions: alcohol, NSAIDs
Beta blockers metoprolol (Toprol XL, Lopressor) carvedilol (Coreg) atenolol (Tenormin)	block beta-adrenergic receptors in the heart (beta$_1$) and blood vessels (beta$_2$) to relax blood vessels	BBW: abrupt discontinuation ADR: dizziness, fatigue, weight gain
*BBW: black box warning **ADR: adverse drug reactions		

Table 7.2. Pharmacological Management of Blood Pressure

Practice Questions

3. Which interventions are likely to be suggested for a 35-year-old patient with diabetes who has good glycemic control and a blood pressure of 135/85?

4. What are the two first-line medications prescribed to patients with diabetes to lower blood pressure?

5. What are the most common side effects of diuretics?

Lipids

Hyperlipidemia—elevated levels of lipids in the blood—increases the risk of atherosclerosis and associated cardiovascular conditions. Patients with diabetes should have a lipid panel done immediately after diagnosis and have their lipid levels checked every four years. Lipid levels should be checked more often for patients at high risk for CVD or those who are already being treated for hyperlipidemia. A lipid panel should include LDL-C, HDL-C, total cholesterol, and triglycerides (see Table 7.3.).

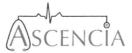

Table 7.3. Lipid Panel		
Lipids		
Low-density lipoprotein cholesterol (LDL-C)	amount of cholesterol carried by LDL molecules; high LDL-C levels associated with <u>increased risk</u> for cardiovascular disease	<100 mg/dL
High-density lipoprotein cholesterol (HDL-C)	amount of cholesterol carried by HDL molecules; high HDL-C levels associated with <u>decreased risk</u> for cardiovascular disease	men: 40 – 50 mg/dL women: 50 – 60 mg/dL
Total cholesterol (LDL and HDL)	combined LDL and HDL cholesterol	<200 mg/dL
Triglycerides	amount of triglycerides (a type of lipid) in the blood; high levels associated with an <u>increased risk</u> of cardiovascular disease	<150 mg/dL

Patients with elevated triglycerides or lower HDL-C should receive counseling on lifestyle management of lipid levels. Specialists should recommend the following lifestyle changes:

- Mediterranean or DASH dietary patterns
- reduction in consumption of saturated and trans fats
- increase in physical activity
- smoking cessation (if appropriate)
- weight loss (if appropriate)

Medications that reduce lipid levels are used to reduce cardiovascular risk for patients with diabetes and hyperlipidemia. The first-line medications for hyperlipidemia are **HMG-CoA reductase inhibitors (statins)**. Second-line drugs may be used in combination with statins for some high-risk patients, particularly those whose lipid levels remain high while on statins. These drugs include the following:

- ezetimibe
- PCSK9 inhibitors (alirocumab and evolocumab)
- bempedoic acid

The types of medications and dosages to manage lipid levels are based on individual cardiovascular risks. General recommendations based on the ADA practice guidelines are described in Table 7.4.

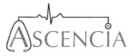

Table 7.4. Pharmacological Management of Hyperlipidemia in Patients with Diabetes

Group	Management	Medications
Low risk: aged <40 years with no other risk factors for CVD	lifestyle interventions	none
Moderate risk: aged <40 years with risk factors for CVD	lifestyle interventions with **moderate-intensity statin therapy**	atorvastatin 10 – 20 mg rosuvastatin 5 – 10 mg simvastatin 20 – 40 mg pravastatin 40 – 80 mg lovastatin 40 mg fluvastatin 80 mg pitavastatin 1 – 4 mg
High risk: ages 40 – 75 with atherosclerosis or other risk factors	lifestyle interventions with **high-intensity statin therapy**	atorvastatin 40 – 80 mg rosuvastatin 20 – 40 mg
Very high risk: patients with 10-year atherosclerotic CVD risk of >20%	lifestyle interventions with maximum-tolerated statin dose and secondary lipid-lowering medication	statin plus ezetimibe or PCSK9 inhibitors

Helpful Hint:

Statin use may damage muscle tissue. Patients on statins should be monitored closely for signs of muscle/joint pain, weakness, and rhabdomyolysis (the breakdown of muscle tissue).

Helpful Hint:

Patients taking atorvastatin, simvastatin, or lovastatin should be advised to avoid grapefruit juice, which increases absorption of these drugs.

Practice Questions

6. A patient on high-intensity statin therapy may be prescribed which two drugs and at what dosages?

7. What is the normal range for triglycerides?

8. Which type of dietary pattern is recommended for patients managing hyperlipidemia?

9. Why would a patient be prescribed ezetimibe?

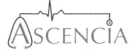

Hepatic Function

The liver functions to maintain glucose homeostasis, so monitoring hepatic or liver function can help detect abnormalities or diseases. **Hepatic function** is the liver's ability to filter blood, detoxify substances, and metabolize proteins/fats. Associations between non-alcoholic fatty liver (NAFLD) disease and type 2 diabetes have been documented. NAFLD, or metabolic dysfunction-association fatty liver disease (MAFLD), can precede or promote the development of type 2 diabetes. Ultrasonography is the preferred imaging technique for monitoring NAFLD. Noninvasive tools, such as liver stiffness measurements, use vibration-controlled or magnetic resonance elastography to identify NAFLD.

There is no general consensus on how to monitor NAFLD, but liver enzyme measurements and ultrasonography are routine every 6 – 12 months after a patient has initiated an intensive lifestyle change. If abnormal enzyme levels are still present, the monitoring continues every 1 – 2 years to obtain a complete blood count and a measurement of lipids, liver enzymes, and fasting glucose. Invasive liver biopsies are considered for patients at increased risk. Normal liver function tests for some enzymes should have an aspartate aminotransferase (AST) less than 31 IU/L (international units per liter) and alanine aminotransferase (ALT) less than 35 IU/L. AST levels for men range from 6 – 34 IU/L and 8 – 40 IU/L for women. ALT levels range from 29 – 33 IU/L for males and about 19 – 25 (IU/L) for females.

Practice Question

10. What are the ranges of AST levels for men and for women that would indicate normal liver function?

Acute Complications: Causes, Prevention, and Treatment

Hypoglycemia and Hypoglycemia Unawareness

Hypoglycemia occurs when plasma glucose levels are abnormally low. People with diabetes (PWD) may experience hypoglycemia for a number of reasons:

- excessive dosages of insulin or glucose-lowering drugs
- increased insulin sensitivity
- comorbid conditions
- exercise or missed meals
- use of alcohol
- acute illnesses or trauma

When hypoglycemia occurs, the neurological and endocrine systems work together to raise glucose levels. The hormones glucagon and epinephrine are released to increase glucose production and reduce the peripheral uptake of glucose. If these steps are ineffective in reversing hypoglycemia, growth hormone and cortisol may also be released. Prolonged hypoglycemia can result in autonomic failure. The common symptoms of hypoglycemia are summarized in Table 7.5.

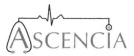

Table 7.5. Causes and Symptoms of Hypoglycemia		
	Autonomic	**Neuroglycopenic**
Cause	The release of epinephrine in response to hypoglycemia activates the sympathetic nervous system.	The lack of available glucose to the brain (neuroglycopenia) causes neurologic dysfunction.
Signs and symptoms	• tremor • palpitations • anxiety • perspiration • nausea • tingling	• weakness • disorientation or confusion • drowsiness • dizziness • loss of consciousness • seizure

While there is not a defined lower limit, a blood glucose (BG) level of <70 mg/dL (level 1 hypoglycemia) generally requires immediate treatment. A level of <54 mg/dL (level 2 hypoglycemia) increases the risk of cognitive dysfunction and death. The presence and timing of hypoglycemic symptoms depend on each person's physiology and clinical history. In some PWD, hypoglycemia symptoms may not appear until even lower BG levels are reached.

Helpful Hint:

Older individuals and patients with long-standing diabetes typically experience more neuroglycopenic symptoms.

Recurrent episodes of hypoglycemia can impair the mechanisms that reverse low BG and prevent the release of hormones, such as epinephrine. Without these mechanisms, many of the symptoms of hypoglycemia are absent, causing **hypoglycemia unawareness** (also called **"impaired awareness of hypoglycemia"**). Because patients have no warning signs that BG levels are low, they are at risk for serious complications, such as neurological dysfunction.

The treatment for hypoglycemia is glucose. Patients can self-manage hypoglycemia using the **15-15 rule**:

- Ingest 15 grams of carbohydrates to raise BG.
- Check BG after 15 minutes.
- Ingest another 15 grams of carbohydrates if BG is still below 70 mg/dL.

Patients should repeat this process until their BG levels are normal. To prevent further drops, they may need to eat a meal or snack after blood sugar levels have returned to normal.

Glucose can be consumed either on its own or in the form of foods that contain simple sugars. The following are common options for treating hypoglycemia:

- glucose tablets or gel
- $\frac{1}{2}$ cup (4 ounces) of juice or normal soda (not diet)
- 1 tablespoon of honey, corn syrup, or sugar
- gumdrops, jelly beans, or hard candies

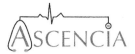

Glucagon can also be administered to quickly increase BG levels. It is available as a nasal spray or an injection (prefilled syringe, auto-injector, and syringe with single-dose vial). All of these alternatives include a fixed dose of glucagon.

If hypoglycemia results in loss of consciousness, a second person or health care professional must deliver glucose, glucagon, or other resuscitative measures. Qualified medical providers can give 25 g of 50% dextrose intravenously (IV) to quickly raise BG. If IV access is not available, a subcutaneous, intramuscular, or nasal administration of glucagon will typically result in a return of consciousness within 15 minutes.

> **Helpful Hint**:
>
> Foods high in fat, like chocolate, take longer to reverse low blood sugar.

Practice Questions

11. Which symptoms of hypoglycemia are caused by a lack of glucose available to the brain?

12. How is the 15-15 rule implemented?

13. What hormone is given as a treatment for hypoglycemia to swiftly raise blood sugar levels?

Hyperglycemia

Treating hyperglycemia is important for managing type 2 diabetes and is necessary to prevent/relieve any acute symptoms and complications. Some acute symptoms of hyperglycemia include the following:

- thirst
- dehydration
- blurred vision
- polyuria
- increased infections.

Acute complications of hyperglycemia include hyperosmolar non-ketotic states and diabetic ketoacidosis (DKA). Hyperglycemic management is also vital for preventing, deferring, or reducing the severity of chronic microvascular complications, e.g., retinopathy.

Causes of hyperglycemia are attributed to eating excess carbohydrates, stress, taking certain medications, and not exercising. People with type 2 diabetes who have abnormal insulin secretion are susceptible to hyperglycemia when insulin shots are not taken regularly.

Prevention of hyperglycemia includes care plans and treatment programs that are tailored and introduced to the individual during diagnosis. Lifestyle changes that include a healthy diet, health education, and exercise are emphasized during diagnosis. If lifestyle interventions cannot achieve ideal glycemic levels, drug treatment or oral agent monotherapy for hyperglycemia is undertaken. Drug therapy ideally addresses pathophysiology, and combinations of different oral glucose-lowering agents are needed to provide efficacy and facilitate therapy. Contraindications and precautions that are associated with each part of pharmacotherapy must be considered. Biguanide metformin is the initial oral glucose-lowering therapy that is selected since it counters insulin resistance and lowers blood glucose; however, if metformin is contraindicated, another class of blood-glucose-lowering therapy is

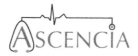

considered. If glycemic targets are not reached, combination therapy can follow, whereby two or three blood glucose-lowering agents are taken. Basal insulin combined with other agents may be combined if glycemic targets are not met.

Practice Question

14. What is the archetypal algorithm for the treatment of hyperglycemia?

Diabetic Ketoacidosis (DKA) and Hyperosmolar Hyperglycemic State (HHS)

Diabetic ketoacidosis (DKA) is a condition characterized by severe hyperglycemia (excessively high BG), **ketosis** (the breakdown of fat for fuel), and acidosis (reduced alkalinity of blood and body tissues). During DKA, elevated serum glucose concentration causes increased urination with significant water loss and electrolyte imbalances.

DKA is most common in people with undiagnosed or ineffectively managed type 1 diabetes (T1D), although it may also occur in people with type 2 diabetes (T2D). It is most often precipitated by infection or failure to use insulin.

Hyperosmolar hyperglycemic state (HHS), also called **hyperglycemic hyperosmolar nonketotic (HHNK) syndrome** is a slow-onset, high-mortality complication of T2D. As with DKA, blood glucose levels become high, resulting in increased urination and hypovolemia (decreased volume of circulating blood). In HHS, insulin production is sufficient to prevent ketoacidosis, which differentiates it from DKA.

Helpful Hint:

Hyperosmolar hyperglycemic state (HHS) is often mistaken for a neurological event because intracerebral dehydration may cause profound central nervous system symptoms, including coma.

Table 7.6. Presentation of DKA and HHS

DKA	HHS
• rapid onset (≤2 days) • increased urination • signs and symptoms of hypovolemia • Kussmaul respirations and fruity breath odor • nausea, vomiting, and abdominal pain • malaise and weakness • decreased level of consciousness (LOC) • elevated BG (>250 mg/dL) • metabolic acidosis • increased serum and urine ketones	• slow onset (≥5 days) • increased urination • signs and symptoms of hypovolemia • rapid, extremely shallow breaths • mild nausea or vomiting • weight loss • malaise and weakness • stupor or coma • severely elevated BG (>600 mg/dL) • no findings of acidosis or ketosis

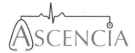

Both DKA and HHS are medical emergencies that require immediate hospitalization for treatment with IV insulin. Patients should be aware of the symptoms of both conditions and know when to seek emergency treatment.

Practice Questions

15. Which mechanism leads patients with severe hyperglycemia to exhibit signs of hypovolemia?

16. A 64-year-old patient newly diagnosed with type 2 diabetes reports weakness, vomiting, and increased urination during the previous three days. A BG check gives a reading of 500 mg/dL. What condition is the patient at risk of developing?

17. What is the priority intervention for patients with DKA or HHS?

Chapter 7 Answer Key

1. The most common target A1C range for people with diabetes (PWD) is <7%.

2. A decrease in the level of 1,5 anhydroglucitol (1,5-AG) indicates that the patient has had periods of hyperglycemia over the previous 2 weeks.

3. This patient should be educated on lifestyle modifications that can lower blood pressure.

4. The first-line medications for lowering blood pressure are angiotensin-converting enzyme (ACE) inhibitors and angiotensin receptor blockers.

5. The most common side effects of diuretics are related to fluid loss from increased urination and include hypotension, weakness, dizziness, and blurred vision.

6. High-intensity statin therapy can include atorvastatin 40 – 80 mg or rosuvastatin 20 – 40 mg.

7. The normal range for triglycerides is <150 mg/dL.

8. The Mediterranean-style dietary pattern and the DASH diet are recommended for patients managing hyperlipidemia.

9. Ezetimibe is prescribed for patients with diabetes who are at very high risk for cardiovascular disease (CVD) and whose lipid levels remain high while on statins.

10. Aspartate aminotransferase (AST) levels range from 6 – 34 IU/L for men and 8 – 40 IU/L for women. ALT levels range from 29 – 33 IU/L for males and about 19 – 25 (IU/L) for females.

11. Hypoglycemia can cause neuroglycopenic symptoms such as weakness, disorientation or confusion, drowsiness, dizziness, loss of consciousness, and seizure.

12. Fifteen grams of carbohydrates will boost blood sugar. Patients should check their BG again in 15 minutes and eat another 15-gram serving of carbohydrates if it is still below 70 mg/dL.

13. Glucagon is administered to swiftly correct hypoglycemia.

14. The general archetypal algorithm for treating hyperglycemia, specifically in people with type 2 diabetes, is as follows:

diagnosis → health education, diet, weight control, exercise → drug treatment or oral agent monotherapy → combination therapy → insulin

15. High serum glucose concentrations lead to increased urination. The excessive water loss causes signs and symptoms of hypovolemia.

16. The patient is showing early signs of hyperosmolar hyperglycemic state (HHS).

17. Patients with diabetic ketoacidosis (DKA) or hyperosmolar hyperglycemic state (HHS) require immediate hospitalization for IV insulin administration.

Chapter 8 - Chronic Complications and Comorbidities

ADA Clinical Practice Screening Recommendations

For young adults with type 2 diabetes, there is an increased risk for several chronic complications and comorbidities

- dyslipidemia
- hypertension
- retinopathy
- nephropathy
- polycystic ovary syndrome (PCOS)
- non-alcoholic fatty liver disease (NAFLD)
- binge eating
- depression

The causes of chronic complications for young adults/teenagers can are numerous and can include the following:

- no longer prioritizing diabetes self-care
- transitioning, emerging adults with diabetes
- having or developing mental health issues
- risk-taking behaviors (e.g., alcohol, drugs)
- an increasing risk of acute complications
- missing screening opportunities

Prevention practices require that PWD are educated on good transitional practices that include screening, meeting, and following up with health care professionals, such as psychiatrists/psychologists and the diabetes specialist. If diabetes complications are not identified early during adolescence, the development of chronic diabetic complications into young adulthood will go untreated and undetected; consequently, other comorbidities may result. Table 8.1. lists ADA screening recommendations and treatments for the various chronic complications seen in diabetic patients.

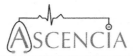
Table 8.1. ADA Screening Recommendations for Chronic Diabetes-Related Complications				
Chronic complication	**Symptoms**	**Screening**	**Treatment**	**Prevention**
Retinopathy (type 1 and 2 diabetes)	• blurred or fluctuating vision • dark/empty areas	• digital imaging (retinal photograph)/retinal examination • dilated fundus examination with a digital fundus camera	• laser photocoagulation surgery • surgical techniques • anti-vascular endothelial growth factor treatment	• glycemic control • blood pressure control
Nephropathy (kidney disease associated with type 1 and 2 diabetes)	• Foot swelling • weight loss • weakness • fatigue • nausea	• glomerular filtration rate (GFR) monitoring • microalbuminuria urine test • GFR blood test • urinary albumin-to-creatine ratio test	• managing hyperglycemia (high blood glucose) • hyperlipidemia • hypertension (blood pressure control) • use of SGLT2 inhibitors	• blood glucose and blood pressure control (ADA does not recommend the use of RAAS inhibitors.)

Practice Question

1. In an attempt to minimize the development of chronic diabetes and other comorbidities, what is the BEST screening method to use to detect complications due to retinopathy?

Vascular Disease

Anatomy and Physiology of the Cardiovascular System

The **cardiovascular system** circulates **blood**, which carries oxygen, waste, hormones, and other important substances dissolved or suspended in liquid plasma. Blood is circulated by the **heart**, which has four chambers, the right and left **atria** and the right and left **ventricles**.

The circulatory system includes two closed loops. In the **pulmonary loop**, deoxygenated blood leaves the heart and travels to the lungs, where it loses carbon dioxide and becomes rich in oxygen. The

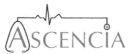

oxygenated blood then returns to the heart, which pumps it through the systemic loop. The **systemic loop** delivers oxygen to the rest of the body and returns deoxygenated blood to the heart.

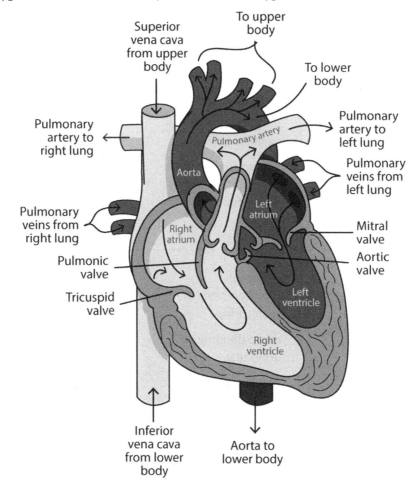

Figure 8.1. The Heart

Blood leaves the heart and travels throughout the body in **blood vessels**, which decrease in diameter as they move away from the heart and toward the tissues and organs. Blood exits the heart through **arteries**, which become **arterioles** and then **capillaries**—the smallest branch of the circulatory system—

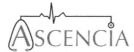

in which gas exchange from blood to tissues occurs. Deoxygenated blood travels back to the heart through **veins**.

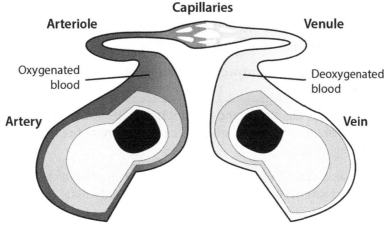

Figure 8.2. Blood Vessels

> **Helpful Hint**:
>
> Blood is supplied to the heart by **coronary arteries:** the **right coronary artery (RCA)**, the **left anterior descending (LAD) artery**, and the **left circumflex (LCX) artery**.

Practice Questions

2. What type of blood vessels carry oxygenated blood away from the heart?

3. In what type of blood vessel does gas exchange occur?

Pathologies of the Cardiovascular System

Cardiovascular disease (CVD) is an umbrella term that describes many conditions that affect the heart and blood vessels:

- hypertension
- atherosclerosis
- myocardial infarction
- stroke
- peripheral vascular disease
- heart failure
- deep vein thrombosis/blood clots

Blood pressure (BP) is the measurement of the force of blood as it flows against the walls of the arteries; it is measured in mm Hg. **Hypotension** is low blood pressure (usually below 90/60 mm Hg).

Chapter 8 - Chronic Complications and Comorbidities

113

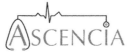

Hypertension is high blood pressure (>120/80 mm Hg). Hypertension often presents with no symptoms but is a significant risk factor for CVD.

Atherosclerosis is a progressive condition in which plaque (composed of fat, white blood cells, and other waste) builds up in the arteries. The presence of advanced atherosclerosis places patients at a high risk for several cardiovascular conditions:

- Arteries may become **stenotic** (narrowed), limiting blood flow to specific areas of the body (e.g., carotid stenosis).

- When a plaque ruptures, the plaque and the clot that forms around it can quickly lead to complete occlusion of the artery (e.g., myocardial infarction) or break off to occlude a smaller vessel (e.g., ischemic stroke).

- Atherosclerosis is also a cause of aneurysms (widened arteries), which weaken arterial walls, increasing the risk of **arterial dissection** or **rupture** (e.g., abdominal aortic aneurysm [AAA]).

A **myocardial infarction** (**MI**, also called a heart attack) is an occlusion of the coronary arteries, which supply blood to the heart. The resulting death of cardiac tissue may lead to dysrhythmias, reduced cardiac output, or cardiac arrest.

Common symptoms of MI include pain or pressure in the chest, jaw, or arm; sweating; nausea or vomiting; and pallor. Some patients, especially women or people with diabetes, may present without chest pain. Patients with MI require immediate medical intervention to restore blood flow to the coronary arteries.

> **Helpful Hint**:
>
> Hyperglycemia alters the tissues that line blood vessels, causing increased buildup of atherosclerotic plaque. This process places people with diabetes at an increased risk of atherosclerosis and related cardiovascular events.

A **stroke**, or **cerebrovascular accident (CVA)**, occurs when blood flow to brain tissue is disrupted. An **ischemic stroke** is the result of a blockage (embolus) in the vasculature of the brain. A **hemorrhagic stroke** is bleeding in the brain, often caused by a ruptured aneurysm. Common symptoms of stroke include severe headache, unilateral weakness or paralysis, and altered mental state.

Atherosclerosis that occurs in peripheral arteries leads to **peripheral arterial disease (PAD)**, also called **peripheral vascular insufficiency**. Symptoms of PAD include pain, tingling, and cramping in the extremities. The **ankle brachial pressure index (ABPI)** (the ratio of ankle systolic pressure to brachial systolic pressure) can be used to assess PAD. An ABPI ratio of <0.80 indicates some level of blockage. An ABPI ratio of <0.30 indicates critical ischemia that requires immediate medical care.

> **Helpful Hint**:
>
> Patients with peripheral neuropathy may not notice common signs of peripheral arterial disease (PAD), such as pain and tingling, so it is important to perform a complete physical assessment during the screening process.

Coronary artery disease (CAD) is narrowing of the coronary arteries and is a significant risk factor for a myocardial infarction. **Heart failure** occurs when either one or both of the ventricles in the heart cannot efficiently pump blood. Because the heart is unable to pump effectively, blood and fluid back up into the lungs (causing pulmonary congestion), or the fluid builds up peripherally (causing edema of the lower extremities).

A **deep vein thrombosis (DVT)** occurs when a blood clot forms within a deep vein, typically in the legs. Left

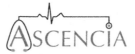

untreated, these blood clots can dislodge and cause a pulmonary embolism. Symptoms include localized pain, unilateral warmth, and edema. Virchow's triad describes the main risk factors for DVT:

- hypercoagulability (e.g., due to estrogen, contraceptive use, or malignancy)

- venous stasis (e.g., bed rest or any other activity that results in decreased physical movement)

- endothelial damage (e.g., damage to the vessel wall caused by hyperglycemia)

CVD is the leading cause of death for patients with diabetes. Chronic hyperglycemia damages large blood vessels, increasing the risk of **macrovascular complications** such as MI, stroke, and PAD. Comorbidities, such as hypertension and hyperlipidemia, can also increase the risk of CVD. The risk of CVD increases the longer a person has diabetes and when diabetes is poorly controlled.

> **Helpful Hint**:
>
> **Nonmodifiable risk factors** for diabetes include genetic predisposition, age, gender, and race/ethnicity. **Modifiable risk factors**—those which a person can change—include obesity, physical inactivity, hypertension, hyperlipidemia, and smoking.

Diabetes also damages smaller vessels, causing **microvascular complications**. This damage can alter blood flow to tissues, including the eyes, kidneys, and nerves, and result in organ dysfunction. Many of the complications discussed in this guide are the result of microvascular damage.

Practice Questions

4. How would a blood pressure of 135/82 mm Hg be classified?

5. Which arteries are affected by a myocardial infarction?

6. What does the ABPI measure?

7. What is the difference between an ischemic stroke and a hemorrhagic stroke?

8. Why does advanced atherosclerosis increase a person's risk for myocardial infarction?

Eye Disease

Anatomy and Physiology of the Eye

The process of sight starts with light passing through the **cornea**, the clear tissue that covers and protects the front of the eye. The light is then filtered by the **iris**, which contracts and dilates to control how much light passes through the **pupil**.

Light travels through the pupil and then the **lens**, which focuses light on the **retina**, the specialized light-sensitive tissue that lines the back of the eye. The **macula** is an area of further-specialized tissue on the retina that is responsible for seeing detail in close objects. Sensory cells in the retina send electronic signals to the brain through the **optic nerve**, which translates the light received into an image.

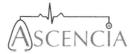

Blood is supplied to the eye by the **central retinal artery** and leaves through the **central retinal vein**. The eye is filled with **vitreous humor**, a jelly-like substance.

Practice Questions

9. Which artery supplies blood to the eye?

10. Which part of the eye senses light and sends signals to the optic nerve?

Pathologies of the Eye

Diabetic retinopathy is characterized by progressive damage to the blood vessels in the retina. The presence and severity of this type of retinopathy is related to the duration of diabetes and level of glycemic control. Signs of retinopathy commonly appear 5 – 10 years after diagnosis; the majority of people who have had diabetes for more than 15 years will have some degree of retinopathy.

The continuum of diabetic retinopathy ranges from mild nonproliferative to proliferative disease. **Nonproliferative retinopathy** begins with microaneurysms in the retina. As the disease progresses, hemorrhages and exudate (exuded matter) in the retina cause swelling and tissue damage.

The growth of new, abnormal blood vessels in the retina marks the progression to **proliferative retinopathy**. These new blood vessels are fragile and prone to bleeding.

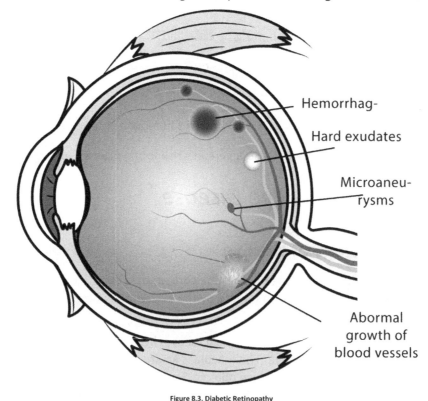

Figure 8.3. Diabetic Retinopathy

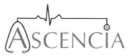

Proliferative retinopathy increases the risk of **retinal detachment**, which occurs when the top layer of the retina is torn away from the underlying tissue. This condition is a medical emergency requiring intervention to preserve sight.

Retinopathy is initially asymptomatic but will affect vision as it progresses. People with retinopathy may see floaters and will eventually develop blurred vision and loss of visual acuity. One of the most frequent reasons for this loss of vision is **macular edema** (swelling of the macula), which can occur with either nonproliferative or proliferative retinopathy.

Management of diabetic retinopathy is initially aimed at slowing the progression of the disease. Patients with lower A1C and BP have lower risks of developing the disease. Once the disease has progressed, it can be managed with drugs to treat swelling and procedures to repair damaged tissue. These procedures, however, only treat the symptoms of the disease. Diabetic retinopathy remains the leading cause of blindness in the developed world.

PWD are at higher risks for other eye conditions, including glaucoma and cataracts. **Glaucoma** is a group of conditions characterized by damage to the optic nerve. The damage is usually caused by increased pressure and swelling within the eye. If left untreated, glaucoma can cause vision loss or blindness.

Cataracts are caused by damage to proteins in the eye that make the lens appear cloudy. It causes blurred, hazy vision. Cataracts are common in older adults, but PWD are at higher risk of developing cataracts earlier in life. For most patients, the cloudy lens can be replaced in a simple outpatient procedure.

Helpful Hint:

Chronic hypertension damages the blood vessels of the eye, leading to **hypertensive retinopathy**. This damage can worsen the retinopathy caused by hyperglycemia in patients with diabetes.

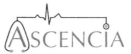

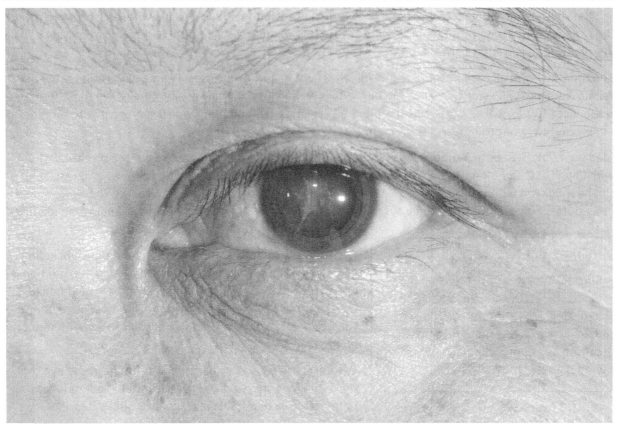

Figure 8.4. Cataract

The American Diabetes Association (ADA) recommends that all PWD have regular screenings by an ophthalmologist for signs of diabetic retinopathy and other eye conditions:

- Patients with T1D should have a thorough eye exam within 5 years of diagnosis.

- Patients with T2D should have a thorough eye exam at the time of diagnosis.

- Patients with T1D or T2D with no signs of retinopathy should have eye exams every 2 years.

- Patients with T1D or T2D with a history of retinopathy should have eye exams at least once a year; exams should be more frequent if the disease is progressing.

- Patients with T1D or T2D should have eye exams prior to becoming pregnant or during the first trimester. These patients should have follow-up exams during pregnancy and for the first year after delivery, depending on the severity of the retinopathy.

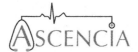

Practice Questions

11. What is the hallmark sign of nonproliferative retinopathy?

12. How often should patients with T2D and no history of diabetic retinopathy have an eye exam?

13. What is the recommended management of early-stage diabetic retinopathy?

14. What eye condition is characterized by clouding in the lens that blurs vision?

Neuropathy

Anatomy and Physiology of the Nervous System

The **nervous system** coordinates the processes and actions of the human body. **Nerve cells**, or **neurons**, communicate through electrical impulses and allow the body to process and respond to stimuli.

The nervous system is broken down into the central and peripheral nervous systems:

- The **central nervous system (CNS)** is made up of the brain and spinal cord.

- The **peripheral nervous system (PNS)** is the collection of nerves that connect the central nervous system to the rest of the body.

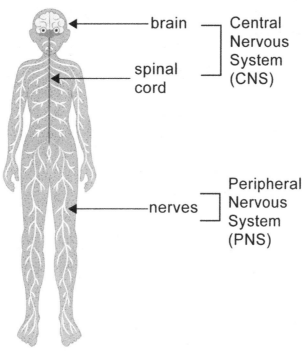

Figure 8.5. The Nervous System

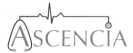

The functions of the nervous system are broken down into the autonomic nervous system and the somatic nervous system:

- The **autonomic nervous system** controls involuntary actions in the body, such as respiration, heartbeat, and digestive processes.

- The **somatic nervous system** is responsible for the body's ability to control skeletal muscles and voluntary movement as well as the involuntary reflexes associated with skeletal muscles. The somatic system includes the sympathetic and parasympathetic systems:

  o The **sympathetic nervous system** is responsible for the body's reaction to stress and induces a "fight-or-flight" response to stimuli (e.g., increased heart rate and BP).
  o The **parasympathetic nervous system** slows the body for rest (e.g., decreased heart rate and BP).

> **Helpful Hint**:
>
> Sympathomimetic drugs mimic epinephrine (adrenaline) and stimulate the autonomic nervous system. They are used to treat shock, allergic reactions, and cardiac arrest. Parasympathomimetic drugs mimic acetylcholine, a neurotransmitter, and activate the parasympathetic nervous system. Nicotine is a naturally occurring parasympathetic compound.

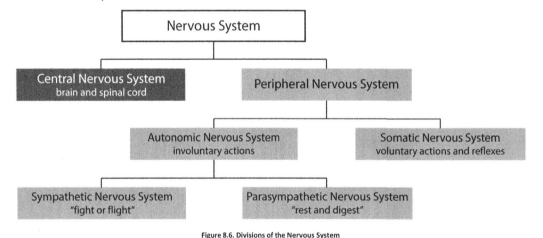

Figure 8.6. Divisions of the Nervous System

Practice Questions

15. The autonomic nervous system is responsible for which functions?

16. What changes are seen in the body when the sympathetic nervous system is activated?

Neuropathies

Diabetic neuropathy is damage to the nervous system seen in PWD. The exact mechanism that causes damage is not known but is likely linked to chronic hyperglycemia.

Diabetic peripheral neuropathy (DPN) affects nerves in the peripheral nervous system, particularly those in the hands, arms, feet, and legs. The condition usually begins in the feet and is typically

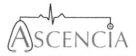

symmetrical. As the condition worsens, sensory loss will extend upward to the calf and start in the hands ("stocking-glove" distribution).

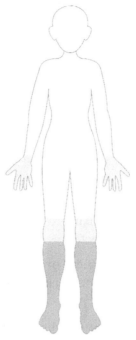

Figure 8.7. Stocking-Glove Distribution of Peripheral Neuropathy

Damage to nerve fibers impairs awareness of position, touch, temperature, and vibration in the affected region; reflexes are also impaired. Symptoms may include pain, burning, or tingling, which is often worse at night. Patients with pain caused by DPN may benefit from drugs such as pregabalin, duloxetine, gabapentin, and tramadol. Because patients with DPN may not notice injuries to the foot, good foot care is also important for these patients. (This topic is covered below in "Lower Extremity Conditions.")

Diabetic autonomic neuropathy (DAN) is damage to nerve tissue in the autonomic nervous system. DAN can affect many physiological processes, including heart rate and rhythm, digestion, urination, sexual function, and sweating. The damage can be diffuse, or it may be confined to one organ. Common autonomic neuropathies are shown in Table 8.2.

Table 8.2. Autonomic Neuropathies

Description	Signs and Symptoms	Management
Cardiovascular autonomic neuropathy (CAN): impairment of autonomic regulation of the cardiovascular system	• tachycardia • exercise intolerance • orthostatic hypotension: lightheadedness, syncope • palpitations	• management of hypertension • management of orthostatic hypotension: increased salt intake, support stockings, fludrocortisone
Gastroparesis:	• bloating and feeling of fullness	• dietary pattern changes (more liquids, less fiber)

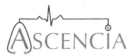

Table 8.2. Autonomic Neuropathies

Description	Signs and Symptoms	Management
delayed gastric emptying that occurs without a gastrointestinal obstruction	• heartburn • upper abdominal pain • nausea and vomiting	• drugs to prevent vomiting and improve motility of GI tract
Urinary dysfunction: diminished capacity to detect a full bladder, leading to overflow incontinence, recurrent urinary tract infections, and a weak urine stream	• trouble urinating • incontinence • s/s of UTI: pain during urination; cloudy, foul-smelling urine	• urination schedule • catheterization • antibiotics to treat UTI
Erectile dysfunction: caused by damage to nerves that control erections	• inability to maintain erection • absence of erection at night and in morning	• PDE-5 inhibitors (e.g., sildenafil [Viagra])
Female sexual dysfunction: reduced hydration of the vaginal mucous membranes due to hyperglycemia, resulting in decreased lubrication	• pain before, during, or after sexual activity (dyspareunia)	• lubrication • topical estrogen
Sudomotor dysfunction: reduced sweat production that can impact thermoregulation and skin health	• anhidrosis (reduced sweat production), often in a stocking-glove pattern • excessive sweating in the upper body • dry, itchy skin	• scrupulous foot and skin care • medications to reduce sweating • lifestyle changes to avoid overheating

Like other diabetic complications, diabetic neuropathy is best managed by tight glycemic control and blood pressure management. Occurrence and severity of DPN and DAN are both correlated with high A1C, hypertension, and hyperlipidemia. The ADA advises screening for neuropathy in all PWD:

- Patients with T1D should be screened within 5 years of diagnosis.

- Patients with T2D should be screened at diagnosis.

- All PWD who do not have symptoms of neuropathy should be screened annually.

- Patients who have prediabetes and neuropathy symptoms should also be regularly screened.

> **Helpful Hint**:
>
> **Silent** (or painless) **myocardial infarction** (MI) occurs when cardiovascular autonomic neuropathy damages nerves in the heart. The resulting lack of symptoms slows diagnosis and delays the provision of MI care.

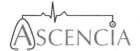

Practice Questions

17. Peripheral neuropathy affects nerves in which areas of the body?

18. The onset of peripheral neuropathy typically occurs in which part of the body?

19. A 54-year-old patient has recently been diagnosed with T2D. When should the patient be screened for peripheral neuropathy for the first time?

20. What type of medication is first-line therapy for erectile dysfunction in patients with diabetes?

21. What is the most common gastrointestinal issue caused by diabetic autonomic neuropathy?

22. What are the most common symptoms of cardiovascular autonomic neuropathy?

Nephropathy

The **renal system** excretes water and waste from the body and is crucial for maintaining the balance of water and salt in the blood (also called electrolyte balance). The main organs of the urinary system are the **kidneys**, which perform several important functions:

- filter waste from the blood

- maintain the electrolyte balance in the blood

- regulate blood volume, pressure, and pH

The functional unit of the kidney is the **nephron**, which is a series of looping tubes that filter the blood. Filtration begins in a network of capillaries called a **glomerulus**, which is located in the **renal cortex** of each kidney. The filtered waste is funneled out of the kidneys into two long tubes called **ureters**. The two ureters drain into the **urinary bladder**. Urine exits the bladder through the **urethra**.

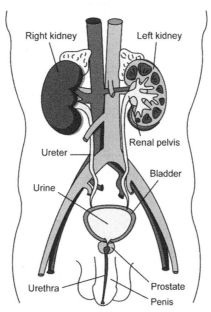

Figure 8.8. The Urinary System (Male)

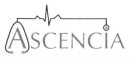

Table 8.3. Kidney Function Tests		
Test	**Description**	**Normal Range**
Urinalysis		
Albumin	protein made by the liver and filtered by the kidneys; high levels indicate renal dysfunction	<30 mg/g
Creatinine	waste product of muscle metabolism; filtered by the kidneys; high levels can indicate renal dysfunction	women: 20 – 275 mg/dL men: 20 – 320 mg/dL
Albumin-to-creatinine ratio (UACR)	unaffected by changes in urine concentration throughout day; increased ratio indicates renal dysfunction	<30 mg/g
Blood Tests		
Estimated glomerular filtration rate (eGFR)	estimated volume of fluid filtered by the renal glomerular capillaries per unit of time; decreased GFR indicates renal dysfunction	women: 90 – 120 mL/min/1.73 m^2 men: 100 – 130 mL/min/1.73 m^2 GFR <60 mL/min/1.73 m^2 is common in adults >70
Blood urea nitrogen (BUN)	by-product of ammonia metabolism; filtered by the kidneys; high serum BUN indicates renal dysfunction	7 – 20 mg/dL
Creatinine	waste product of muscle metabolism; filtered by the kidneys; high serum creatinine indicates renal dysfunction	0.6 – 1.2 mg/dL
BUN-to-creatinine ratio	increased ratio indicates dehydration, acute kidney injury, or gastrointestinal bleeding; decreased ratio indicates renal dysfunction	10:1 – 20:1

Chapter 8 - Chronic Complications and Comorbidities

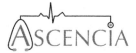

Practice Questions

23. What are the functions of the kidneys?

24. Where does most of the filtration occur in the kidneys?

Diabetic Nephropathy

Diabetic nephropathy (DN) is damage to the kidneys caused by diabetes. It is the primary cause of **chronic kidney disease (CKD)**—progressive dysfunction of the kidneys lasting more than 3 months. An estimated 20% – 40% of patients with diabetes have DN.

Diabetic nephropathy damages nephrons in the kidneys, reducing their ability to filter proteins and other waste from the body. Screening for kidney dysfunction uses the urine albumin-to-creatinine ratio (UACR), which can be tested with spot urinalysis. A UACR of ≥30 mg/g twice in 6 months is defined as **albuminuria** and indicates renal dysfunction.

Patients with CKD are initially asymptomatic since the kidneys compensate for tissue damage. As the disease progresses, fluid builds up in the body. Serious complications can follow, including peripheral edema, pulmonary edema, and congestive heart failure. Waste also builds up in the blood (uremia), which can have profound effects throughout the body. **End-stage renal disease (ESRD**, also called **kidney failure**) is the last stage of the disease; patients with ESRD require dialysis or a kidney transplant to survive. The stages of CKD are measured by glomerular filtration rate (GFR), which steadily declines as renal function decreases:

- stage 1: >90 mL/min
- stage 2: 60 – 89 mL/min
- stage 3: 30 – 59 mL/min
- stage 4: 15 – 29 mL/min
- stage 5: <15 mL/min (ESRD)

Patients with diabetic nephropathy will experience a decline in renal function; however, attentive management can significantly slow progression of the disease. Patient management of DN includes the following:

- tight glycemic control (A1C ≤7.0%)
- aggressive blood pressure control (<130/80 mm Hg)
- limiting protein intake to 0.8 to 1.2 g/kg/day (severely restricting protein intake is not recommended)

The ADA recommends annual screenings for all people who have had a diagnosis of type 1 diabetes for at least five years. For patients diagnosed with type 2 diabetes, the ADA recommends annual screenings starting at the time of diagnosis.

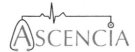

Practice Questions

25. What albumin-to-creatinine ratio indicates albuminuria?

26. How many grams of protein should a person with overt nephropathy eat per kilogram of body weight?

27. What serious medical conditions are caused by fluid buildup due to CKD?

Lower Extremity Problems

Damage to the feet is a serious concern for PWD. A combination of peripheral neuropathy, peripheral arterial disease, and/or impaired healing can cause mild injuries to worsen quickly. Foot ulcers and complications are linked to increased hospital readmissions, prolonged inpatient stays, and elevated morbidity and mortality for PWD. Common foot conditions include ulcers, bullae, Charcot foot, and calluses.

Diabetic foot ulcers are the most serious foot complication seen in PWD. (See "Dermatological Problems" below for information about ulcers.) Patients with poorly treated foot ulcers will eventually require hospitalization and, possibly, amputation.

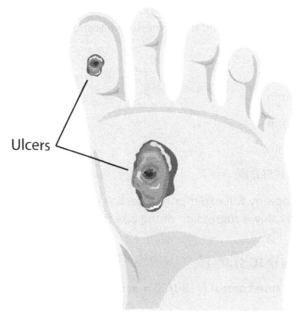

Ulcers

Figure 8.9. Diabetic Foot Ulcer

Diabetic bullae are noninflammatory, blistering lesions on the legs, foot, and toes. Bullae might be a few millimeters or many centimeters in size. They are generally mild but may create slight burning sensations. Bullae caused by diabetes are treated conservatively: the intention is to lessen discomfort and reduce the possibility of subsequent infection.

Charcot foot (also called Charcot arthropathy) is the progressive deterioration of the soft tissues, joints, and bones of the foot or ankle. Bones can break as they deteriorate, and deformity can occur when the

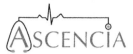

joints in the foot or ankle dislocate and collapse. Deformities can also increase the risk of ulcerations over bony areas.

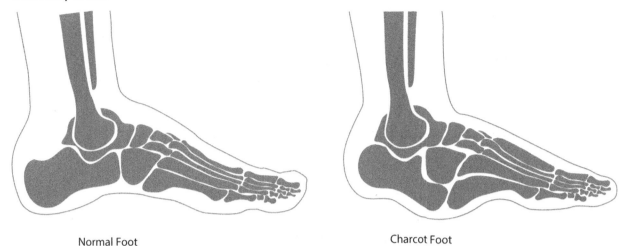

Normal Foot   Charcot Foot

Figure 8.10. Example of Deformity Caused by Charcot Foot

Deformity or a lack of sensation in the foot can allow abnormal pressure to persist undetected by the patient. Skin cells respond to this pressure with increased keratinization, causing a **callus** to form. Patients with calluses are more likely to develop foot ulcers and subsequent infections.

Practice Questions

28. Where are diabetic bullae most frequently found on the body?

29. What medical disorder causes progressive deformation of the bones, joints, and soft tissue in the feet?

30. How do calluses develop?

Foot Care

The ADA recommends that PWD have a comprehensive foot exam annually. Patients with peripheral neuropathy or a history of foot issues should have their feet examined at every visit. PWD who exhibit atypical findings during the thorough foot examination should be referred to a foot care specialist. A comprehensive assessment includes the following elements:

- **inspection:** complete visual inspection of the foot, looking for skin conditions (e.g., ulcers, redness), bone and joint deformity, and balance/gait

- **vascular evaluation:** assessment for reduced pedal pulses, decreased skin temperature, and thin/blueish skin

- **checks for protective sensation loss:** pinprick, vibration, touch, or monofilament tests to check for reduced sensitivity to sensation and loss of ankle reflexes

- **radiographic imaging:** scan for structural foot deformities, gas in soft tissues, and foreign objects

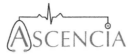

People with Type I and II diabetes with acute painful neuropathy experience burning pain on the plantar part of the feet. Diabetes care and education specialists should teach patients about preventive foot care and how to assess their own feet. Patient self-care techniques include the following:

- trimming toenails to the curve of the toe, smoothing jagged edges using a file, and leaving cuticles intact

- washing feet in lukewarm water and thoroughly drying, especially between the toes

- moisturizing feet (except between toes) to avoid cracks in dry skin

- wearing comfortable shoes customized to fit underlying foot malformations

- changing socks and shoes daily

- avoiding going barefoot

- performing regular visual assessments of the feet

Practice Questions

31. What tests are used to determine whether protective feeling has been lost?

32. How should patients with diabetes trim their toenails?

33. How should patients with diabetes be instructed to wash their feet?

Chapter 8 - Chronic Complications and Comorbidities

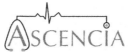

Anatomy and Physiology of the Skin

The **integumentary system** refers to the **skin**—the largest organ in the body—and related structures, including the hair and nails. Skin is composed of three layers:

- The **epidermis** is the outermost layer of the skin. This waterproof layer has no blood vessels and acts mainly to protect the body.

- Under the epidermis lies the **dermis**, which consists of dense connective tissue that allows skin to stretch and flex. The dermis contains blood vessels, glands, and hair follicles.

- The **hypodermis** is a layer of fat below the dermis that stores energy (in the form of fat) and acts as a cushion for the body. The hypodermis is sometimes called the **subcutaneous layer**.

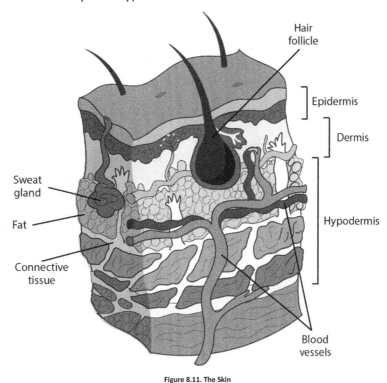

Figure 8.11. The Skin

Practice Questions

34. What is the outermost layer of the skin called?

35. What is the function of the hypodermis?

Dermatological Problems

The skin can be affected by diabetes in much the same way as other organs. Damage to blood vessels can cause damage to skin tissues, and impaired healing increases the risk of skin infection. Specific skin conditions commonly seen in PWD include ulcers, diabetic dermopathy, acanthosis nigricans, diabetic thick skin, and skin infections.

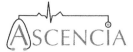

Ulcers are open wounds surrounded by inflamed, damaged, or necrotic tissue. PWD can have ulcers on any area of the skin, but the most common location is the foot. Ulcers are usually the result of injury or pressure (e.g., poorly fitting shoes) that damages tissue. Healing is impaired by hyperglycemia and poor circulation.

There are a number of systems for staging ulcers, including the Wagner, University of Texas, and WIfI (wound [W], ischemia [I], and foot infection [fI]) classification systems. Ulcers are generally staged based on the progression of tissue damage (from epidermis through to bone), perfusion to the area, and the presence of infection. Treatment of ulcers may include debridement of dead tissue, antibiotics, and wound closure.

Diabetic dermopathy is the presence of small, round; pink, reddish, or brown areas on the skin. It is usually seen on the arms, thighs, or lower legs. It is believed to be caused by damage to blood vessels in the skin. Dermopathy caused by diabetes typically does not require treatment.

Acanthosis nigricans is a condition with characteristic dark, velvety bands of discolored skin in body creases or folds. It is frequently seen in people who are overweight or obese and is linked to increased insulin resistance. Acanthosis nigricans cannot be treated, but the discoloration can fade with improved glycemic control.

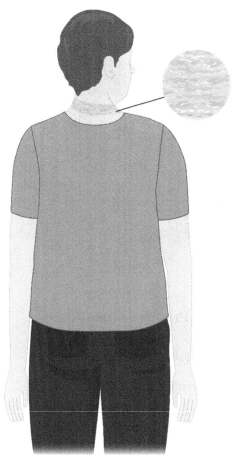

Figure 8.12. Acanthosis Nigricans

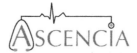

Poorly controlled diabetes can lead to **diabetic thick skin**. Areas of thickened, waxy skin usually appear on the hands or feet, where it is known as digital sclerosis, and may spread to the arms, shoulders, or back. The condition does not present a serious health threat, but it may constrict movement.

Practice Questions

36. What skin condition is characterized by dark, velvety bands of discolored skin in body creases or folds?

37. Where are ulcers most commonly seen on PWD?

38. What treatment is recommended for diabetic dermopathy?

Infection

Anatomy and Physiology of the Immune System

The human **immune system** protects the body against bacteria and viruses that cause disease. The system is composed of two parts: the innate system and the adaptive system.

The **innate immune system** includes nonspecific defenses that work against a wide range of infectious agents. This system includes physical barriers that keep out foreign particles as well as organisms and cells that attack invaders.

Barriers to entry are the first lines of defense in the immune system. These include the skin, mucus, and native bacteria that outcompete invaders. Pathogens, however, sometimes breach these barriers and enter the body, where they attempt to replicate and cause an infection. When this occurs, the body mounts a number of nonspecific responses. The body's initial response is **inflammation**, which increases blood flow to the infected area. This increase in blood flow increases the presence of **white blood cells**, also called **leukocytes**, which destroy invaders or infected cells.

The second part of the immune system is the **adaptive immune system**, which "learns" to respond only to specific invaders. Pathogens contain **antigens**, foreign molecules that trigger the adaptive immune system. Once triggered, the system creates and deploys specialized cells that respond to the antigen that started the process.

In the cell-mediated response to antigens, **T cells** destroy any cell that displays an antigen. In the antibody-mediated

> **Helpful Hint**:
>
> Memory B cells and T cells are the underlying mechanisms behind vaccines, which introduce a harmless version of a pathogen into the body to activate the body's adaptive immune response.

response, **B cells** are activated by antigens and go on to produce antibodies. **Antibodies** bind to specific antigens and destroy the cells that contain them. Memory B cells are created during infection, allowing the immune system to respond more quickly if the infection appears again.

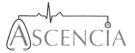

Practice Questions

39. How is the innate immune system different from the adaptive immune system?

40. Breast milk contains antibodies from the mother's immune system. How do these antibodies protect breastfeeding infants from infection?

Infections in People with Diabetes

People with type 1 and 2 diabetes have higher risks of infection, such as yeast infections of the genitourinary tract and pulmonary or respiratory infections:

Elevated blood glucose can lead to respiratory bacterial infections, such as Legionella pneumonia. The genitourinary tract consists of organs of the urinary and reproductive systems, which include the ureters, kidneys, urethra, bladder, and reproductive organs.

Females with diabetes who have hyperglycemia are susceptible to vaginal Candidiasis, or inflammation of the vagina and vulva since high blood glucose will allow yeasts to thrive in a glucose-rich environment. The body can excrete excess sugar in the urine, sweat, and mucus, and yeast will grow more so in warm and moist environments where these bodily fluids are present. Severe genitourinary infections are painful and irritating and can interfere with sexual intercourse. Fungal infections such as *Candidiasis*, caused by *Candida albicans* or the Candida species, will penetrate the mucosal lining of the vagina resulting in inflammation, burning sensations, irritation, and swelling. Skin discoloration can also occur.

Males with diabetes who have a yeast infection or Candidiasis will experience swelling and pain in the groin area. Irritation, a scaly rash, and itching will occur under the foreskin and head of the penis. White-like discharges can occur.

Acute Infections can be treated with suppositories (in women) and antifungal creams. An oral dose of 150 mg of fluconazole or terconazole can be applied intravaginally for 3 – 7 days. For complicated infections that include patients who have recurrent infections or are immunosuppressed, extended treatment regimens are implemented. Oral treatment with 150 mg of fluconazole every three days or Intravaginal azole therapy for 7 days can be administered. Optimizing blood glucose levels in men and women with diabetes can reduce the chance of reinfection. Medical studies have indicated an increased risk of genitourinary infections with the use of SGLT-2 inhibitors; high dosages of dapagliflozin also lead to an increased risk.

Practice Question

41. What is the correlation between blood sugar levels and yeast infections?

Dental and Gum Diseases

The center of a tooth contains **pulp**, a combination of blood vessels and nerves. The pulp is covered and protected by **dentin**, a mineralized tissue that is harder than bone. The dentin is covered in **enamel**, another mineralized tissue that protects the inside of the tooth. The visible portion of the tooth is the **crown**.

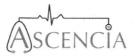

The portion of the tooth below the gumline (i.e., not visible) is the **root**. The root sits within the **alveolar process**, a part of the jaw bone. The alveolar bone and the tissues that anchor teeth within it form the **periodontium**. Other parts of the periodontium include **cementum** (which covers the dentin in the root), **gingiva** (the soft tissue of the gums), and ligaments.

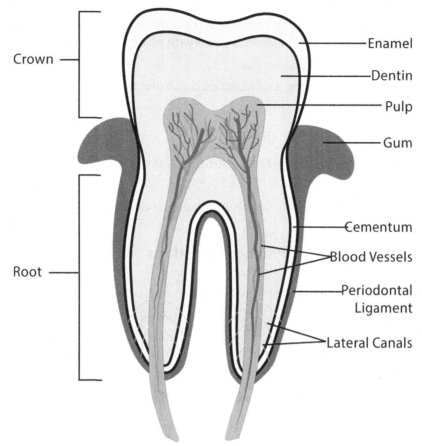

Figure 8.13. Anatomy of a Tooth

Dental and gum diseases are both highly correlated with diabetes. The relationship moves in in both directions. PWD are more likely to develop dental conditions, particularly periodontal disease. Dental diseases can also worsen glycemic control by making it harder for patients to chew and eat healthy foods.

The following common dental issues are seen in people with diabetes:

- **Caries** (cavities) is tooth decay caused by bacteria that gradually break down tooth enamel. These bacteria coat the mouth and teeth in a soft, sticky layer called **plaque**. Because the bacteria that cause caries feed on sugar, foods that are high in sugar can worsen tooth decay.

> **Helpful Hint**:
>
> Liquid foods, such as smoothies, often contain high levels of sugar. Patients who rely on liquid foods due to dental issues will likely see large spikes in BG levels.

- **Periodontal disease** is inflammation of the periodontal tissues (the gums, alveolar bone, and tissues that attach the tooth to bone). Like tooth decay, periodontal disease is caused by the bacteria in plaque. Periodontal disease is the most common cause of tooth loss in adults.

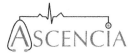

- **Gingivitis** is inflammation of the gums. If left untreated, the inflammation can progress to other tissues in the periodontium and lead to tooth loss.

- **Xerostomia** (dry mouth) is more common in patients with T2D. Because saliva helps protect the mouth from harmful bacteria, a lack of saliva production can increase the risk of dental disease.

Because diabetes can depress the immune system, PWD are more prone to **oral mucosal diseases** such as fungal infections (e.g., candidiasis) and ulcers. People with diabetes should be educated on proper oral hygiene measures:

- brushing teeth twice a day using a soft-bristled brush and fluoride toothpaste

- flossing once a day

- using fluoride rinses, gels, or varnish

- minimizing consumption of sugary foods, particularly those that stick to the teeth (e.g., caramel)

- visiting the dentist every 6 months (more if periodontal disease is present)

> **Helpful Hint**:
>
> Fluoride is a mineral that strengthens tooth enamel and prevents decay.

Practice Questions

42. Which anatomical structures are part of the periodontium?

43. What causes caries?

44. How often should people with diabetes and no history of periodontal disease visit the dentist?

Other Comorbidities

Thyroid Disease

The **thyroid**, a butterfly-shaped gland located in the lower neck, controls the body's metabolism by secreting thyroid hormone. Thyroid hormone has two forms: **thyroxine (T4)** and **triiodothyronine (T3)**. The level of these hormones can be used to assess thyroid function, as described in Table 8.4.

Table 8.4. Thyroid Function Tests		
Test	**Description**	**Normal Range**
Thyroid stimulating hormone (TSH)	TSH is produced by the anterior pituitary gland. High TSH indicates hypothyroidism; low TSH indicates hyperthyroidism.	0.5 – 5.0 mIU/L
T4	T4 is produced by the thyroid gland. High levels indicate hyperthyroidism; low levels indicate hypothyroidism.	5.0 – 12.0 µg/dL

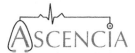

Table 8.4. Thyroid Function Tests		
Test	**Description**	**Normal Range**
T3	T3 is produced by the thyroid gland. High levels indicate hyperthyroidism; low levels indicate hypothyroidism.	80 – 220 ng/dL

There is a strong correlation between diabetes and thyroid disorders. Patients with T1D are at particularly high risk, with estimates of 15% – 30% of such patients having both diabetes and autoimmune-induced thyroid disorders. Dysfunction in the thyroid can lead to hypo- or hyperthyroidism. The symptoms and treatments for these are summarized in Table 8.5.

Table 8.5. Thyroid Disorders		
	Hyperthyroidism	**Hypothyroidism**
Description	The thyroid overproduces thyroid hormone, which speeds up metabolism.	The thyroid underproduces thyroid hormone, which slows down metabolism.
Symptoms	<ul><li>pounding heart and increased heart rate</li><li>trouble concentrating, anxiety, or irritability</li><li>weight loss</li><li>breathlessness</li><li>diarrhea</li><li>muscle weakness or tremors</li></ul>	<ul><li>slow heartbeat and hypotension</li><li>fatigue</li><li>depression</li><li>weight gain</li><li>feeling cold even when others are feeling warm</li><li>constipation</li></ul>
Treatment	thioamides (e.g., carbimazole and propylthiouracil), which prevent the thyroid from overproducing hormones	synthetic thyroid hormones (levothyroxine)

Helpful Hint

The symptoms of hyperthyroidism and hypoglycemia are very similar. Patients with thyroid issues should always check their blood glucose (BG) levels before treating hypoglycemia.

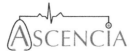

Practice Questions

45. Which type of diabetes places patients at the highest risk of developing thyroid disorders?

46. Low BG mimics which thyroid condition?

Sleep Apnea

Sleep apnea is a sleep disorder characterized by bouts of whole or partial airway obstruction during sleep. The presence of sleep apnea is strongly correlated with T2D, particularly for patients who are obese. Symptoms of sleep apnea include the following:

- loud snoring
- gasping for breath while sleeping
- periods of not breathing while sleeping
- awakening with a dry mouth or painful throat
- fatigue and sleepiness during the day

> **Helpful Hint:**
> Sleep disruptions from apnea can alter glucose metabolism and increase insulin resistance, making glycemic control more difficult.

Mild sleep apnea can be managed with lifestyle changes, including weight loss, positional changes at night, and the use of a mouthpiece to open the airway. Moderate to severe sleep apnea is treated with **continuous positive airway pressure (CPAP)**. With this treatment, a machine forces air through a face mask the patient wears while sleeping; the force of the air keeps the airway open. The use of a CPAP machine increases daytime alertness, improves memory and cognitive function, improves glucose and insulin sensitivity during the night, and reduces the incidence of dawn phenomenon (high blood sugar in the morning).

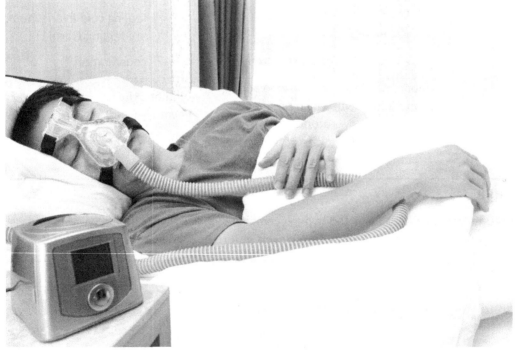

Figure 8.14. CPAP Machine

Chapter 8 - Chronic Complications and Comorbidities

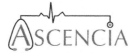

Practice Questions

47. What are the symptoms of sleep apnea?

48. What is the treatment for moderate to severe sleep apnea?

Polycystic Ovary Syndrome

Polycystic ovary syndrome (PCOS) is caused by the dysregulation of androgens (e.g., testosterone) and estrogen. Women with PCOS present with symptoms of hyperandrogenism and the following metabolic disorders:

- thinning hair on scalp and excessive hair growth on the body

- acne

- obesity

- missed or irregular periods

- infertility

- ovarian cysts

PCOS is correlated with T2D. PCOS increases insulin resistance and leads to hyperinsulinemia. Women with PCOS should be regularly screened for diabetes.

Management of PCOS includes lifestyle changes to promote weight loss and improve insulin sensitivity. Patients may also require oral contraceptives (to maintain regular periods) or androgen blockers to alleviate symptoms.

Practice Questions

49. Which type of diabetes is more common in women with polycystic ovary syndrome?

50. What are common symptoms of PCOS?

Depression

An association and bidirectional relationship is present between diabetes and depression. Depression is a risk factor associated with diabetes, and adults who are depressed have a 37% increased chance of developing type 2 diabetes. People with type 2 diabetes were found to have a positive association with depressive symptoms; consequently, the ability of PWD to achieve optimal glycemic management can be more difficult, which can decrease their quality of life.

Depression is a common comorbid condition that can lead to erectile dysfunction (in men) and sexual dysfunction (in women). Treatment studies indicate that improving glucose levels can reduce depressive symptoms.

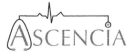

Practice Question

51. How are depression and diabetes related?

Celiac Disease

Celiac disease, an autoimmune disease, causes inflammation and/or damage to the small intestine when exposed to gluten. While the disease is present in genetically predisposed people with HLA-DQ2/DQ8 haplotypes, other predispositions may be present. There is an association between celiac disease and type 1 diabetes; however, there is no link between type 2 diabetes and celiac disease. Approximately 6% of people with type 1 diabetes have celiac disease. Untreated celiac disease can make patients more susceptible to hypoglycemia since the small intestine cannot absorb nutrients, such as sugar. Strict gluten-free diets that are followed early on and that avoid wheat, rye, and barley can reduce the chances of developing autoimmune disorders. Comorbidities such as neuropathy, gastrointestinal issues, and weight gain may be due to diabetes or celiac disease.

Practice Question

52. How does celiac disease, if left untreated, lead to hypoglycemia?

Obesity

People with obesity will often experience weight bias, stigma, and discrimination. Weight bias includes the idea that obesity is a lifestyle choice and that people who are obese lack motivation and discipline. Exposure to weight bias and stigma, which can occur in the workplace, can lead to weight gain and exercise avoidance, thereby affecting physical and mental health.

Weight stigma is associated with anxiety, obesity, and the risk of type 2 diabetes. One study indicated that 40% of patients with celiac disease were overweight and 13% were obese, which places patients at higher risk for developing type 2 diabetes. Processed gluten-free products are of concern since they have a higher glycemic index with more fat and less protein, which can contribute to weight gain and obesity.

Practice Questions

53. How does weight bias affect a person's risk of developing type 2 diabetes?

Chapter 8 Answer Key

1. Dilated fundus examination through digital imaging is a technique that enlarges the pupil to examine the fundus of the eye. Diabetic retinopathy causes irreversible damage to the retinal blood vessels, which can lead to blindness. Examination of the fundus, or interior of the eye, will allow the physician to detect any abnormalities of the blood vessels.

2. Arteries carry oxygenated blood away from the heart.

3. Gas exchange from blood to tissues occurs in the capillaries.

4. A blood pressure of 135/82 mm Hg is classified as hypertension.

5. A myocardial infarction is occlusion of the coronary arteries.

6. The ankle brachial pressure index (ABPI) is the ratio of ankle systolic pressure to brachial systolic pressure; it is used to assess peripheral arterial disease (PAD).

7. An ischemic stroke is caused by occlusion of a blood vessel in the brain. A hemorrhagic stroke is bleeding in the brain.

8. Atherosclerosis is the buildup of plaque in blood vessels. When a plaque ruptures, the plaque and the clot that forms around it can quickly lead to complete occlusion of a coronary artery.

9. The central retinal artery supplies blood to the eye.

10. The retina senses light and sends signals to the optic nerve.

11. The hallmark sign of nonproliferative retinopathy is microaneurysms in the retina.

12. Patients with type 2 diabetes (T2D) and no history of diabetic retinopathy should have an eye exam every two years.

13. The recommended management of early-stage diabetic retinopathy is maintaining low A1C levels and blood pressure to slow progression of the disease.

14. Cataracts are characterized by clouding in the lens that blurs vision.

15. The autonomic nervous system controls involuntary actions in the body, including respiration, heartbeat, and digestive processes.

16. The sympathetic nervous system activates the "fight-or-flight" response, which includes an increased heart rate and increased blood pressure (BP).

17. Peripheral neuropathy affects peripheral nerves, particularly those in the hands, arms, feet, and legs.

18. Typically, peripheral neuropathy starts in the feet.

19. Patients diagnosed with type 2 diabetes (T2D) should be immediately screened for neuropathy.

20. PDE-5 inhibitors are first-line therapy for erectile dysfunction in patients with diabetes (PWD).

21. The most common gastrointestinal issue caused by diabetic autonomic neuropathy is gastroparesis.

22. The most common symptoms of cardiovascular autonomic neuropathy are tachycardia, exercise intolerance, orthostatic hypotension, and palpitations.

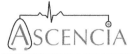

23. Kidneys filter waste from the blood; maintain the electrolyte balance in the blood; and regulate blood volume, blood pressure (BP), and pH.

24. Most of the filtration in the kidneys occurs in a network of capillaries called a glomerulus.

25. An albumin-to-creatinine ratio of ≥30 mg/g measured twice in 6 months indicates albuminuria.

26. The American Diabetes Association (ADA) advises people with diabetes and overt nephropathy to limit their protein intake to 0.8 to 1.2 g/kg/day.

27. Buildup of fluid secondary to chronic kidney disease (CKD) can cause peripheral edema, pulmonary edema, and congestive heart failure.

28. Diabetic bullae most frequently appear on the legs, feet, and toes.

29. Charcot foot, or Charcot arthropathy, causes progressive deformation of the bones, joints, and soft tissue in the feet.

30. Skin cells respond to persistent abnormal pressure on the foot by producing more keratin, which develops into a callus.

31. Examinations using monofilament, vibration, touch, or pinprick can be used to test for the lack of protective feeling.

32. Toenails should be trimmed to the curved shape of the toe. All sharp edges should be smoothed off, and cuticles should not be cut.

33. Patients with diabetes should be instructed to wash their feet in lukewarm water and dry them thoroughly, particularly between the toes.

34. The outermost layer of the skin is the epidermis.

35. The hypodermis is a layer of fat below the dermis that stores energy (in the form of fat) and acts as a cushion for the body.

36. Acanthosis nigricans is the presence of dark, velvet-like bands of discolored skin in body creases or folds.

37. Most ulcers in patients with diabetes (PWD) occur on the foot.

38. Diabetic dermopathy does not usually require treatment.

39. The innate immune system defenses work against a wide range of infectious agents, while the adaptive immune system responds to specific antigens it has encountered before.

40. Antibodies attach to antigens and destroy pathogens that cause infection. Because the mother and child have likely been exposed to the same pathogens, the mother's antibodies can help protect the infant from such pathogens.

41. High levels of blood sugar provide a glucose-rich environment in which yeasts can thrive, thereby increasing the chances of such infections in patients with diabetes.

42. The periodontium is composed of the alveolar bone, cementum, gingiva, and ligaments.

43. Caries is caused by bacteria in the mouth that gradually break down tooth enamel.

44. The ADA recommends that people with diabetes and no history of periodontal disease visit the dentist every 6 months.

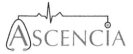

45. Patients with type 1 diabetes (T1D) are at the highest risk of developing thyroid disorders.

46. Low blood glucose (BG) symptoms mimic hyperthyroidism.

47. The symptoms of sleep apnea include loud snoring, gasping for breath while sleeping, periods of not breathing while sleeping, awakening with a dry mouth or painful throat, and fatigue or sleepiness during the day.

48. The treatment for moderate to severe sleep apnea is a continuous positive airway pressure (CPAP) machine.

49. Patients with polycystic ovary syndrome (PCOS) are often insulin resistant, which increases their risk for type 2 diabetes (T2D).

50. Common symptoms of polycystic ovary syndrome (PCOS) include thinning hair on the scalp and excessive hair growth on the body, acne, obesity, missed or irregular periods, and infertility.

51. Diabetes and depression have a bidirectional relationship—there is a connection between the two. Depression is a risk factor associated with diabetes; adults with depression have a 37% increased chance of developing type 2 diabetes.

52. When left untreated, celiac disease prevents the small intestine from absorbing nutrients, which makes people with the disease more susceptible to hypoglycemia.

53. Experiencing weight bias—the idea that people have chosen obesity and/or are lazy and lack discipline—can trigger anxiety in people with obesity. This leads to a ripple effect wherein the toll on the person's mental health leads them to avoid exercise, which in turn leads to more weight gain, which can lead to further mental and physical health complications, such as the development of diabetes.

Chapter 9 - Problem-Solving

Sick Days

During an acute illness, the body releases hormones that raise BG levels and increase insulin resistance. The combination of these effects can raise BG to dangerous levels. If not monitored closely, PWD are at risk for severe hyperglycemia during acute illnesses. PWDs should use the following guidelines to manage sick days:

- Continue to take insulin and antidiabetic agents as directed by the provider, even when the patient is sick.
    - During an illness, BG levels can rise to dangerous rates even if the patient is not eating; insulin doses should never be skipped and may need to be increased.
    - For tighter glycemic control, patients who take antidiabetic agents for T2D may need to switch to insulin during severe illnesses.
- Drink enough calorie-free liquids to stay hydrated, especially with symptoms such as excess urination, vomiting, and diarrhea.
- Check glucose levels every 2 – 4 hours.
- Check urine ketone levels every 4 hours to monitor for DKA if the patient uses insulin.
- Maintain a **sick box** with supplies, including BG and ketone testing strips, antidiabetic agents, glucose, and a BG monitor with extra batteries.
- Contact the patient's provider or seek urgent care for symptoms of DKA, persistent vomiting or diarrhea, and/or persistent fever.

Helpful Hint:

Patients may be reluctant to start taking insulin when they are sick. Remind patients that starting insulin does not mean staying on it for the long term; they can transition back to their regular antidiabetic agents after the illness is resolved.

Practice Questions

1. How do acute infections or illnesses affect blood glucose levels?

2. The flu is going around. Several patients with type 2 diabetes who use basal insulin have asked if they need to take their insulin if they are too sick to eat. How should the specialist respond?

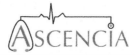
Surgery and Other Procedures

Psychosocial factors will influence the lifestyle and medical outcomes of a person with diabetes. Therefore, practicing personalized/patient-centered care requires problem identification, communication and interactions, and intervention with the person with diabetes. The ADA/EASD supports person-centered diabetes care to improve the patient's engagement in self-care behaviors since self-care can improve clinical outcomes and enhance patient education. Diabetes care should focus on the quality of life and function, disease control, tailored treatment recommendations for an individual's unique situation, balancing the benefits and risks of treatment, promoting self-management, and agreement on an individualized care plan.

Advancements in surgery for type 2 diabetes can reduce comorbidities and lead to a better quality of life. While surgery has some risks that include nutritional deficiency, surgical complications, and psychological symptoms, these operations have been fine-tuned over several decades with a 0.6 – 1.1% mortality rate. Surgical risks are generally smaller compared to a pharmacological approach to glycemic treatment.

Bariatric surgery can reduce hunger and support the body's ability to achieve a healthy weight. When considering the benefits or risks of surgery, a surgeon will review and discuss different surgical procedures with the patient and determine if surgery is appropriate. PWD who are considering bariatric surgery are recommended to complete mental health assessments before surgery. Following surgery, patients should be assessed regularly to ensure that psychiatric symptoms do not interfere with weight loss or lifestyle changes.

Practice Question

3. How are person-centered care and clinical outcomes connected?

Schedule Changes

Travel

Caring for diabetes requires close monitoring and management of blood glucose levels. Travel can disrupt normal care routines, placing patients at risk for hypo- and hyperglycemia. Patients should follow these guidelines when traveling:

- Discuss travel plans with a provider and get necessary documentation (e.g., signed prescriptions).

- Check glucose levels frequently during travel.

- Pack twice as much of the antidiabetic agent(s) as needed for the trip.

- Be careful with testing supplies and antidiabetic agents; pack them safely and do not store them in hot or cold areas (e.g., airplane baggage compartment, trunk of car).

- Move around during flights and car trips to lower the risk of blood clots.

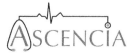

- Be aware of the differences in available insulin strengths in other countries. Outside the US, insulin is typically available in strengths U-40 or U-80 and requires a different syringe and dosage compared to the common U-100 available in the US.

- Adjust insulin doses and timing when crossing time zones.

- Travel with snacks, beverages, or glucose to manage hypoglycemia.

- Always wear medical identification.

Changes to schedules or shifts will impact self-care management for people with diabetes. For instance, patients who have irregular schedules or night shifts will face additional challenges controlling their diabetes and lifestyles. Overnight shift work is common in fields such as health care and law enforcement. While the benefit of irregular schedules may include better pay, research has indicated that shift work can either worsen diabetes or put people at higher risks of developing type 2 diabetes. In general, the CDC recommends eating at normal times, keeping track of sleep, avoiding caffeine at the end of shifts, and exercising. Taking medication consistently and monitoring blood sugar is vital for diabetes self-management.

Practice Question

4. What is the standard insulin strength outside of the United States?

Religious, Spiritual, and Cultural-Related Schedule Changes

Many PWD who manage their diabetes will rely on their religious and/or spiritual beliefs as a means of support. Many studies have indicated a strong connection between diabetes self-care practices and religious/spiritual beliefs. Some of these self-care practices that have impacted diabetes management include the adoption of healthy food choices, optimal medication practices or routines that include consistent glucose monitoring, and increased physical activity. Diabetes management programs have been introduced to churches, mosques, or other houses of worship. These programs incorporate strategies that involve the communication of diabetes care through newsletters, which provide additional resources and information for the prevention of diabetes. Religious fasting for Muslims, Christians, Hindus, and other groups is an important life aspect; therefore, these groups must follow specific health education programs that help individuals keep their glucose levels on target.

Certain cultures will have different attitudes towards physical activity, which can present a barrier to managing diabetes. For example, some cultures face barriers to physical activity that include a lack of time due to expectations of having long work hours and time-consuming career commitments. Structured education programs that enhance self-care and the promotion of physical activity programs are needed interventions in some ethnic minority groups but can be challenging to launch due to low levels of recruitment. In one study, churches in low-income neighborhoods in New York City included nutrition education and fitness activities that statistically changed the participant's dietary habits by eating less fast food.

Practice Question

5. How do different cultural and religious beliefs affect diabetes management?

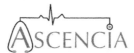

Assistive and Adaptive Devices

Poor or low vision is a problem present in people with diabetic retinopathy or a history of diabetes where glucose levels remain high. Ways to improve everyday activities include using anti-glare eyewear or incorporating brighter lights at home. Magnification devices are another way to improve quality of life. They include a stand magnifier, handheld magnifier, reading glasses magnifier, clip-ons, and tele-microscopic glasses. Diabetes-specific devices also include audio glucometers, lancets, continuous glucose monitors, and insulin pens. Audio glucometers read glucose numbers aloud, and continuous glucose monitors provide audio alters for preset high or low glucose levels. Insulin pens make audible clicking noises during insulin delivery.

Practice Question

6. What is the name of the device that provides audio and real-time glucose alerts without the use of a lancet?

Substance Use

Decades of research has shown that smoking tobacco is linked to poor health outcomes. In addition to causing lung disease, smoking raises blood pressure, causes microvascular damage, and increases the risk of CVD and stroke. Because PWD are already at higher risk of CVD, smoking is particularly dangerous for these patients.

Patients who smoke should be offered help with **smoking cessation** if they have indicated they are motivated to quit. Patients may choose from a number of methods to quit smoking, including tapering or choosing to quit all at once (going "cold turkey"). There are a number of support interventions that may help:

- nicotine patches, gum, and sprays
- counseling
- support groups
- prescription medications

Table 9.1. Prescription Medications for Smoking Cessation	
Drug	**Description**
Varenicline (Chantix)	blocks nicotine receptors to make smoking less pleasurable and dulls the effects of withdrawal; may cause gastrointestinal symptoms and mood changes
Bupropion (Zyban, Wellbutrin)	antidepressant that reduces cravings for nicotine; may include side effects such as dry mouth, trouble sleeping, GI symptoms, and mood changes
Nortriptyline	antidepressant that may help reduce cravings for nicotine; may include side effects such as tachycardia, dry mouth, GI symptoms, and mood changes

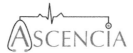

Table 9.1. Prescription Medications for Smoking Cessation	
Drug	**Description**
Clonidine	sedative and antihypertensive medication that may help reduce cravings for nicotine; may include side effects such as drowsiness, dizziness, dry mouth, and constipation

Nicotine is addictive, and many patients will find smoking cessation difficult. The specialist should be sensitive to patients' needs and work with them to build personalized quitting plans. Research has shown that a combination of counseling and medication is most effective. Group counseling in particular increases the chance patients will successfully quit.

The care specialist may also practice harm reduction by guiding patients toward lower-risk options, such as smoking fewer cigarettes or using a personal electronic cigarette. While these options still carry risk, they may be more attainable for the patient.

Substances besides nicotine can also affect PWD. For example, the consumption of two or more amounts of drip-filtered caffeinated coffee was associated with better glucose tolerance and lowering the risk of type 2 diabetes; however, short-term metabolic studies of patients with type 2 and gestational diabetes who consume caffeine have shown a lower insulin sensitivity but increased glucose concentrations. People with type 1 diabetes showed decreased hypoglycemic episodes when consuming caffeine.

Erectile dysfunction (ED) is a common obstacle in men with diabetes, and it can worsen with the use of specific substances. In a systematic review and meta-analysis of 145 studies that included nearly 89,000 men with diabetes, there was an ED prevalence of about 53%. Men with diabetes are more likely to be taking medications or drugs that can impair their ability to have erections. Some medications or substances that are associated with ED include antihypertensives, antidepressants, antipsychotics, hormones, prescription drugs such as statins, and drugs such as marijuana and opiates. Antihypertensives such as beta-blockers, thiazide diuretics, and aldosterone receptor blockers/antagonists have been reported to have the greatest risks to erectile function, while alpha-blockers have the least amount of risks. Specialists should advise men with diabetes who have ED to consider oral therapies, which include oral agents such as phosphodiesterase 5-inhibitors (PDE5); examples include sildenafil, tadalafil, vardenafil, avanafil, mirodenafil, and udenafil. Sildenafil, in particular, has been highly effective in the treatment of ED, with a nearly 70% success rate.

Practice Questions

7. People with type 1 diabetes would likely benefit from coffee consumption. Is this statement true or false?

8. What side effects might be experienced by patients taking Chantix?

9. What interventions are the MOST effective in helping patients quit smoking?

Chapter 9 Answer Key

1. During infections, the body releases hormones that increase blood glucose levels.

2. The specialist should tell the patients that they need to continue taking insulin even if they are not eating.

3. Self-care is known to improve clinical outcomes and enhance patient education, which is why the ADA/EASD supports this type of approach to care.

4. Outside of the United States, insulin is typically available in 40 or 80 units per mL strength (U-40 or U-80).

5. Some religious traditions include periodic fasting, which can have an effect on blood sugar levels, and some cultures place greater emphasis on careers and other time-consuming commitments. Still other cultures face barriers to self-care strategies, such as physical activity, due to location and other factors. In response to some of these challenges, various religious institutions have begun diabetes management and education programs, which have been shown to have a positive effect on the participants.

6. Continuous glucose monitors (CGMs) will monitor blood glucose in real time and alert the patient when glucose levels are high or low. The CGM uses a small sensor that is inserted below the skin of the belly or arm. The electrode sensor will then measure the glucose levels within the tissue, a technique that has nearly replaced the need for finger pricking.

7. People with type 1 diabetes will benefit from the consumption of caffeinated coffee, which leads to decreased instances of hypoglycemic episodes.

8. Side effects of Chantix include gastrointestinal (GI) symptoms and mood changes.

9. A combination of counseling—particularly in a group setting—and medication has been shown to be the most effective way to help people stop smoking.

Chapter 10 – Living with Diabetes and Prediabetes

An effective **diabetes care plan** aligns with medical practice standards and is personalized to meet the individual needs of the patient. The plan is developed by an interdisciplinary team that includes all medical providers involved in the patient's care. If patients also have an active role in their care and are considered members of the care team, they will be more likely to meet goals built around their personal values, preferences, and abilities.

Treatment Plans

Goals of a Treatment Plan

The two main goals of a care plan are to delay or prevent complications from diabetes and to improve quality of life. To accomplish these goals, the care plan should incorporate both lifestyle and pharmacological interventions to help the patient maintain glycemic control.

The care plan should cycle through a process of assessment and modification to take into account the patient's successes and needs. This cycle includes the following steps:

1. **Assess the patient, including factors that affect choice of treatment:** Patients should receive a thorough assessment that includes a health history and physical exam. The specialist should take special note of factors that may influence treatment planning:

- the patient's financial resources
- the patient's ability to follow a medication regimen
- the patient's motivation
- depression or other mental health issues experienced by the patient
- the patient's tolerance for medication side effects
- the patient's health literacy and familiarity with technology

> **Helpful Hint**:
>
> Care planning should center on the patient. On the CDCES exam, the correct answer is usually the one that prioritizes the patient's needs and concerns.

2. **Work collaboratively with patients to set goals:** The care team should work with patients and their families and caregivers to develop the care plan. This process should empower the patients to make decisions.

3. **Implement the plan:** The specialist should ensure that patients understand their care plans and have access to the resources they need to implement them.

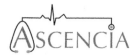

4. **Provide ongoing monitoring and support:** Patients should be seen at least every 3 months. Patients who are not making progress may require more frequent contact. The health care team should regularly monitor the following factors:

- glycemic status

- emotional status

- medication adherence and side effects

- physical markers (e.g., weight, blood pressure, lipids)

5. **Review and modify the care plan:** The care plan should be reviewed at least once a year to make needed changes. Revisions to the plan should be agreed on by both the patient and the care team.

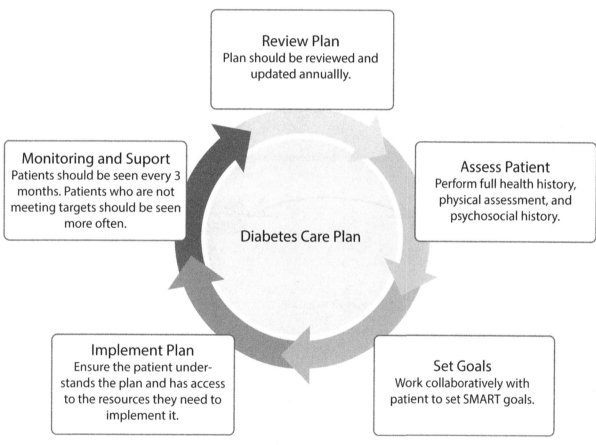

Figure 10.1. Patient-Centered Care Plan Cycle

Practice Questions

1. What are the TWO main goals of a management plan?

2. After a care plan has been implemented, what is the next step the health care team should take?

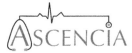

Treatment Plan Evaluation, Documentation, and Follow-up

A diabetes care team consists of a group of health professionals who will provide support to the patient with diabetes. The team may include the certified diabetes care and education specialist (CDCES), diabetes physician, dietitian, and psychologist. The team will exchange information, advice, and education in order to develop a tailored patient plan to help support the patient with diabetes. Importantly, the health care team must have access to previous patient records so that the team is fully aware of the patient's medical history, background, and experience with diabetes. Documents or forms, such as "Questions to Ask" consist of checklists for patients to use to determine which questions to ask their physicians and steps to follow to provide better self-care and metabolic management. The **kaleidoscope model of care** is a novel method for tailoring an individual's plan for care and is designed to be revised based on specific factors. The model is dynamic and can adapt to the needed range of care.

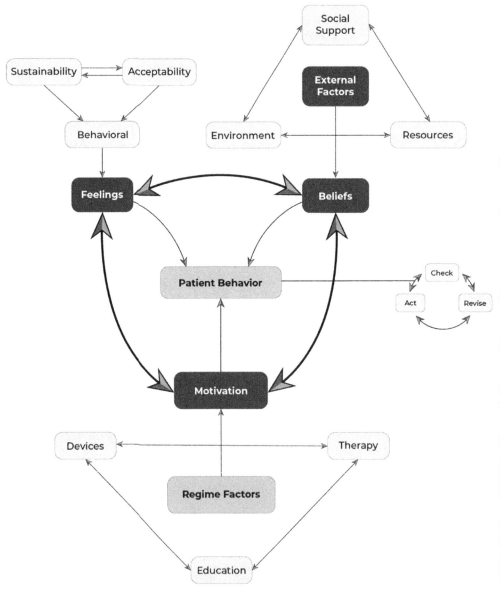

Figure 10.2. The Kaleidoscope Model of Care

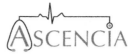

Physicians should provide PWD with copies of letters written about them and should encourage the patients to develop questions about treatment recommendations. PWD must be kept aware of the next steps in their care plans and know whether additional investigation is needed for specific treatments. In a process called **care planning**, the individual and specialist will discuss and review management plans through joint dialogue, discussion, and listening. This process will enhance relationships and partnerships.

Practice Question

3. Briefly describe the kaleidoscope model of care.

Special Populations

Pediatric Patients and Child Development

Type 1 diabetes (T1D) is the most common type of diabetes seen in pediatric patients, with diagnosis usually occurring between the ages of 3 and 5 or 10 and 14 (during puberty). However, the incidence of pediatric type 2 diabetes (T2D)— usually diagnosed during adolescence—is growing, particularly in Black and Hispanic/Latino populations. Pediatric patients with T2D generally show a faster decline in beta cell function and develop complications faster than adults with T2D.

> **Helpful Hint**:
>
> Diabetes is extremely rare in infants and toddlers. Less than 2% of pediatric diabetes patients are under 3 years old.

Management of diabetes in pediatric patients presents unique challenges to both caregivers and diabetes care and education specialists. Everyone involved in the child's care must be ready to adjust goals and interventions as the child passes through developmental stages.

Table 10.1. Special Considerations for Pediatric Patients with Diabetes	
Age Group	**Special Considerations**
Infant (1 month – 1 year) and **Toddler** (1 – 3 years)	• Set loose blood glucose (BG) targets to prevent hypoglycemia, which can damage the growing central nervous system. • Adjust insulin doses frequently to account for rapid growth. • Use rapid-acting insulin after meals/snacks (instead of preprandial administration) so that the dose can be adjusted for the amount of food consumed. • Rotate injection sites frequently and use short, thin needles. • Check BG to distinguish hypoglycemia from common behavioral issues. • Monitor BG overnight, if necessary. • Provide support for parents, who may feel intense anxiety or guilt.
Preschool 3 – 5 years	• Adjust insulin doses frequently to account for rapid growth.

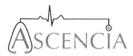

Table 10.1. Special Considerations for Pediatric Patients with Diabetes	
Age Group	**Special Considerations**
	• Use rapid-acting insulin after meals/snacks (instead of preprandial administration) so that the dose can be adjusted for the amount of food consumed. • Gradually increase the child's involvement in care (e.g., let the child complete small tasks such as turning on the meter or creating a visual logbook that can be completed with stickers). • Engage the child's imagination with medical play but be aware that preschoolers may develop fantastical scenarios around medical care (e.g., "If I stop eating then I won't have to get any more shots."). • Develop comprehensive care plans for other caregivers, including day care teachers and babysitters.
Elementary school 5 – 11 years	• Children ages 5 – 11 still require frequent adjustments to insulin doses. • Children will begin to be influenced by peers, which may make them less likely to adhere to care plans (e.g., snacking at parties, unwillingness to test in a school setting). • Engagement in physical activity, such as PE or a sports program, requires a testing and insulin plan. • Work with school personnel to provide education and develop a comprehensive care plan. • Continue to encourage independence and a growing involvement in care.
Younger adolescents 11 – 14 years	• Hormonal fluctuations that accompany puberty lead to insulin resistance, which necessitates frequent adjustments to insulin regimen. • Young adolescents may become self-conscious and attempt to hide their diabetes conditions and care from peers. • Young adolescents may want to take more control of care but might not yet be able to fully manage independently; continue to allow the child to manage more aspects of care. • Provide counseling to patients struggling with anger, depression, or body issues.
Older adolescents 14 – 18 years	• Teens may develop eating disorders or skip insulin doses to lose weight. • Provide education for relevant issues, including sexual health, driving, and the use of alcohol/drugs.

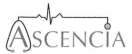

Table 10.1. Special Considerations for Pediatric Patients with Diabetes	
Age Group	**Special Considerations**
	• Begin the transition to fully independent care by letting teens make their own care decisions and interact independently with the care team.

> **Helpful Hint**:
>
> Bed-wetting can be a sign of hyperglycemia in toilet-trained children.

Practice Questions

4. The parent of a 3-year-old with diabetes has trouble providing the correct insulin dose because the child eats an unpredictable amount of food at dinner. What intervention should the specialist suggest?

5. A 16-year-old with T1D has an A1C of 8.5% and has recently lost 10 pounds. The patient claims to be injecting insulin correctly as noted in logbooks. What is the most likely explanation the specialist should consider?

6. Why do the insulin regimens of young adolescents with diabetes need to be adjusted frequently?

Blood Glucose Management for Pediatric Patients

Pediatric patients, particularly the very young, are at risk for hypoglycemia due to a number of factors:

- unpredictable eating and activity patterns

- frequent changes in insulin needs related to rapid growth

- difficulty in providing consistent care across different childcare settings

Young children may not recognize the signs of hypoglycemia or be able to communicate them to a caregiver. Caregivers may also mistake the signs of hypoglycemia for typical childhood development issues (e.g., moodiness, altered speech or motor skills).

To lower the risk for hypoglycemia, BG targets are kept looser for pediatric patients, particularly for the very young. Pediatric patients typically have an A1C target of <7%. This value might be increased to <7.5% for patients with a history of hypoglycemia or patients who do not have access to necessary glucose monitoring or insulin delivery technology.

BG targets are adjusted by age. General guidelines for these targets are shown in Table 10.2.

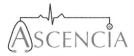

Table 10.2. BG Targets for Pediatric Patients with Diabetes (mg/dL)			
	Age <6	**Ages 6 – 12**	**Ages 13 – 18**
Fasting	80 – 180	80 – 180	70 – 150
Preprandial	100 – 180	90 – 180	90 – 130
Bedtime	110 – 200	100 – 180	90 – 150

Pediatric patients with T1D require insulin. Most children require 0.5 – 0.8 units/kg per day. This number will increase during puberty, when dose requirements may be as high as 1.5 units/kg per day. Typically, between 50% and 60% of insulin will be basal.

Pediatric patients with T2D should receive pharmacological interventions similar to those for adult patients. Metformin should be initiated at diagnosis if not contraindicated. Patients with severe hyperglycemia may also require basal and/or bolus insulin.

Pediatric patients with diabetes should be screened for common complications. A summary of the screening recommendations from the American Diabetes Association (ADA) is provided in Table 10.3.

Table 10.3. Screening Recommendations for Pediatric Patients with Diabetes		
	Type 1 Diabetes	**Type 2 Diabetes**
Thyroid issues	• Screen at diagnosis. • Follow up every 1 – 2 years.	
Celiac disease	• Screen at diagnosis. • Follow up within 2 years and then every 5 years.	
Hypertension	• Screen at diagnosis. • Follow up at every visit.	
Dyslipidemia	• Screen at diagnosis. • Follow up at 9 – 11 years and every 3 years if LDL <100 mg/dL.	• Screen at diagnosis. • Follow up annually.
Nephropathy, retinopathy, and neuropathy	• Screen at diagnosis. • Follow up annually. • Follow up every 2 years for retinopathy for T1D.	
Nonalcoholic fatty liver disease	N/A	• Screen at diagnosis. • Follow up annually.

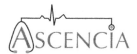

Table 10.3. Screening Recommendations for Pediatric Patients with Diabetes		
	Type 1 Diabetes	**Type 2 Diabetes**
Obstructive sleep apnea and polycystic ovary syndrome		• Screen at diagnosis. • Follow up at every visit.

Practice Questions

7. What is the typical A1C target for most pediatric patients with diabetes?

8. What is the honeymoon period of type 1 diabetes?

9. How often should pediatric patients with type 1 diabetes be screened for nephropathy?

Older Adults

Providers should be aware of how diabetes specifically affects older adults. Patients older than 65 are physiologically different from younger patients and may have had diabetes and/or complications for a long period of time. Their care goals will also be different, as treatment benefits must be weighed against quality of life and life expectancy. All of these issues must be accounted for when developing an individualized plan for older adults.

The following physiological changes, caused by aging, can significantly affect diabetes care:

- a reduction in fluid volume that increases the risk of dehydration

- changes in the gastrointestinal system, including changes to taste, reduction in saliva, and reduced motility, all of which can affect nutritional intake

- changes in the liver and kidneys that can alter how drugs are metabolized

- changes in eyesight, hearing, mobility, and cognitive function that can affect self-care

- a higher likelihood of having comorbidities, including kidney and cardiovascular disease

- a higher likelihood of having care complicated by polypharmacy

- a higher risk of cognitive decline and dementia

- a higher likelihood of falling, which can lead to serious injury

Care plans for older adults must help patients manage BG levels while also navigating the complex issues described above. Management of hyperglycemia in older adults is generally less aggressive than in younger patients. Older adults are at higher risk for hypoglycemia; they are more likely to require insulin and may also face more self-care challenges. Hypoglycemia is especially dangerous for older patients because it increases the risk of falls and may

Helpful Hint:

Medical treatments that affect red blood cell turnover, such as transfusions or erythropoietin-stimulating agents, are more common in older adults. These treatments can make A1C results unreliable, so providers may need to rely on blood glucose monitoring to make treatment decisions.

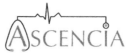

worsen cognitive decline. The ADA's BG monitoring guidelines for older patients are summarized in Table 10.4.

Table 10.4. Blood Glucose Targets for Older Adults with Diabetes		
Patient Health Status	A1C Target (%)	Fasting or Preprandial BG Target (mg/dL)
Healthy with few complications	<7.0 – 7.5	80 – 130
Moderately complex with multiple comorbidities or moderate cognitive impairment	<8.0	90 – 150
Very complex with end-stage chronic illness or severe cognitive impairment	Do not use A1C. Care should focus on avoiding hypoglycemia and symptomatic hyperglycemia.	100 – 180

Antidiabetic agents for older adults should be managed carefully. Older adults with diabetes often benefit from a simplified regimen that includes both fewer medications and less-frequent doses.

Metformin is the recommended first-line treatment for T2D in older adults. Drugs that increase the risk of hypoglycemia, including sulfonylureas, should be used cautiously. Insulin may be prescribed as needed, but dosages should be tailored to the patient's abilities and lifestyle. Older adults may struggle with the physical and cognitive requirements of a complex insulin routine. Often, a single dose of long-acting basal insulin is the best option.

Older adults should be monitored closely for cognitive, sensory, and functional deficits. These changes may impact the patient's ability to care for themselves. Older patients should also be regularly assessed for depression—isolation and lack of social support are common problems for older adults.

Practice Questions

10. What is the ADA's recommended target A1C for a 67-year-old patient who lives independently and does not have coexisting chronic conditions or any functional or social concerns?

11. What family of medications should be used cautiously in older patients with type 2 diabetes with a history of hypoglycemia?

12. Why are older patients at a higher risk of dehydration?

Other Populations

Patients with end-stage renal/kidney disease can have a better quality of life with a kidney transplant; however, they can also be at risk of developing posttransplant diabetes mellitus (PTDM). Some patients diagnosed with PTDM had diabetes before the transplant. About 10 – 30% of patients who have received a kidney transplant are diagnosed with PTDM. Complications associated with PTDM are similar to those associated with PWD, but complications such as strokes or kidney disease can develop more quickly. Treatments for PTDM must consider possible drug interactions, kidney function, and side

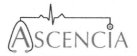

effects. For example, since the kidney is unable to recover fully after a transplant, the use of antidiabetic agents that are eliminated by the kidneys may not be advisable.

At least 40% of kidney transplant candidates have a BMI over 30, so weight management education for the recovering patient is an important part of preventing PTDM.

After the transplant, insulin therapy is needed to manage hyperglycemia, especially since the patient will be taking high-dose immunosuppressants. In addition to blood glucose monitoring, the patient may require enteral nutrition. PTDM patients can then transition to multiple-daily insulin injections once they have stable nutritional regimens. Some patients may be candidates for oral hypoglycemic medications. Metformin and sulfonylureas are commonly utilized for PTDM but may carry some risks. GLP-1 agonists and sodium-glucose cotransporter-2 inhibitors must be used with extreme caution.

Practice Questions

13. Why is insulin therapy needed after a kidney transplant?

Pregnancy

Preconception Planning

Ideally, patients with preexisting diabetes who plan to become pregnant should receive preconception care. This care includes all standard education for pregnancy (e.g., taking folic acid; avoiding alcohol, nicotine, and recreational drugs). Patients with diabetes should also be educated on the following risks associated with hyperglycemia during pregnancy:

- spontaneous abortion

- preeclampsia

- fetal anomalies

- neonatal conditions (e.g., hyperbilirubinemia)

To help avoid these outcomes, patients should maintain tight glycemic control leading up to pregnancy. Providers should also swap or modify medications that may be harmful during pregnancy (e.g., statins, ACE inhibitors).

> **Helpful Hint**:
>
> The most common drugs used to treat hypertension during pregnancy are methyldopa (which decreases sympathetic nervous system activity) and labetalol (a beta blocker).

Pregnancy can increase the risk of diabetic retinopathy. PWD who are planning to become pregnant should have an eye exam before pregnancy to establish a baseline and then at least once a trimester during pregnancy.

Practice Question

14. A patient with type 2 diabetes currently takes lisinopril, atorvastatin, and chlorothiazide. Which of these medications should be discontinued before pregnancy?

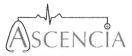

Pregnancy and Delivery

Tight glycemic control should be maintained throughout pregnancy. Table 10.5. summarizes the ADA's recommendations for patients who are pregnant.

Table 10.5. Blood Glucose Targets During Pregnancy			
Type 1 and Type 2 Diabetes		**Gestational Diabetes**	
Blood Glucose Monitoring	**Continuous Glucose Monitoring**	**Blood Glucose Monitoring**	
<ul><li>fasting: 70 – 95 mg/dL</li><li>one-hour postprandial: 110 – 140 mg/dL</li><li>two-hour postprandial: 100 – 120 mg/dL</li></ul>	<ul><li>target range: 63 – 140 mg/dL</li><li>The target time in, above, and below range does not change.</li></ul>	<ul><li>fasting: <95 mg/dL (5.3 mmol/L)</li><li>one-hour postprandial: <140 mg/dL (7.8 mmol/L)</li><li>2-hour postprandial: <120 mg/dL (6.7 mmol/L)</li></ul>	
An A1C of <6% is correlated with better health outcomes during pregnancy; however, because of the physiological changes that occur during pregnancy, A1C is not a reliable indicator of blood glucose or the risk of hyperglycemic complications.			

Patients with T1D will need to adjust their insulin doses regularly throughout pregnancy. Insulin requirements typically drop in the first trimester due to increased insulin sensitivity and glucose uptake by the fetus. Patients will be at risk of hypoglycemia if insulin doses are not adjusted down.

> **Helpful Hint**:
>
> Due to changes in red blood cells during pregnancy, A1C is slightly lower for most people during pregnancy.

Between weeks 16 and 36, blood glucose levels will steadily rise if insulin doses are not increased. During the third trimester, patients will require higher amounts of insulin than were needed before pregnancy. Patients who are pregnant can develop diabetic ketoacidosis (DKA) at lower BG levels, so patients should be educated on DKA prevention and symptoms.

> **Helpful Hint**:
>
> Patients with type 1 or type 2 diabetes should be prescribed low-dose aspirin during pregnancy to lower the risk of preeclampsia.

The preferred treatments for T2D during pregnancy are lifestyle modifications and insulin. Many T2D medications, including metformin and sulfonylureas, easily pass through the placenta and should not be used during pregnancy. Patients should receive medical nutrition therapy and be encouraged to exercise.

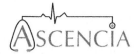

Practice Questions

15. What is the current medical treatment recommendation for a person with type 2 diabetes who becomes pregnant?

16. What is the fasting glucose target range for patients with type 1 diabetes who are pregnant?

17. What happens to a patient's insulin needs during the first trimester of pregnancy?

Postnatal Care

Patients who require insulin during pregnancy should be closely monitored immediately after giving birth. Insulin sensitivity increases quickly after the placenta is delivered, and insulin needs will drop dramatically. Insulin needs should return to pre-pregnancy levels 1 – 2 weeks after delivery.

Patients with gestational diabetes mellitus (GDM) should have a fasting 75 g oral glucose tolerance test at 4 – 12 weeks postpartum to evaluate for persistent diabetes. (GDM can be a presentation of preexisting diabetes that was not previously diagnosed.) All patients diagnosed with GDM should be screened for diabetes every 1 – 3 years. These patients should also be encouraged to adopt lifestyle modifications that reduce the risk of developing type 2 diabetes.

> **Helpful Hint**:
>
> Most antidiabetic agents, including insulin and metformin, are safe to take while breastfeeding.

Breastfeeding is encouraged for all mothers, including those with diabetes; however, PWD should be mindful that the increased use of glucose during lactation reduces their insulin needs. These patients should check BG levels before and after nursing.

Practice Question

18. A patient with type 1 diabetes is about to give birth. How will this patient's insulin needs change immediately after delivery?

Safety

Sharps Disposal

All used needles need to be disposed of safely. Sharps disposal units can be purchased online or in medical supply stores. Alternatively, patients can dispose of needles in containers that include a lid, such as a plastic container or one made of another shatterproof material. To help identify the contents, the container should be clearly labeled "Medical Sharps." A sharps disposal unit should also be used when traveling.

> **Helpful Hint**:
>
> For sanitation and safety purposes, used needles cannot be recycled and should not be placed in recycling bins.

Medical Identification

All PWD should wear or carry some type of medical identification that states that they have diabetes. A medical ID card or bracelet will alert medical personnel or bystanders

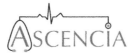

during a medical emergency so that the appropriate care can be provided quickly. Information about the person's diabetes can also be stored in the emergency section of a person's mobile phone.

Driving

Episodes of hypoglycemia that occur while driving can endanger both the driver and other people on the road. People who use insulin should always check BG levels before driving, and they should not drive if they are hypoglycemic. If PWD experience symptoms of hypoglycemia, they should pull over immediately. A supply of snacks or glucose should be kept in the car in case of hypoglycemic episodes. Every state has specific laws and regulations that govern driver's license restrictions for people with diabetes.

Practice Questions

19. What is the best place to dispose of used needles?

20. What should patients with type 1 diabetes always do before driving?

Social and Financial Considerations

Health Insurance

Insurance companies act as financial intermediaries between patients and medical care providers. The consumer pays the insurance company a **premium**—a regular, predetermined amount of money. In return, the insurer covers some part of the financial costs of the consumer's medical care. The types of services covered and the amount the insurance company will pay are determined by the insurance plan.

Most health care in the United States is provided through **managed care organizations (MCOs)**. MCOs seek to control costs while maintaining access to high-quality health care by managing patients' use of medical services. MCOs work toward these goals by using the following methods:

- contracting with providers so their members can access services at a discounted rate

- requiring patients to use only specific providers

- requiring referrals or preapproval for specialized medical care

- easing access to lower-cost preventive care

- limiting the amount paid for specific services

- denying payment for services they determine are not medically necessary

> **Helpful Hint**:
>
> Caring for PWD often requires working closely with insurance companies. Specialists may be required to assist with submitting insurance claims, sending referrals, and acquiring pre-authorization for tests and procedures.

MCOs also minimize the amount they pay for a patient's medical care by sharing the cost of care with the patient. In addition to the cost of their premium, patients share the cost of their medical expenses through payments referred to as co-pays, deductibles, and coinsurance:

- **Co-pays** are set payments that patients pay each time they seek medical care. For example, patients might have to pay a $15 co-pay when they see their medical provider.

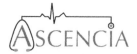

- A **deductible** is a set amount that patients must pay in a given year before the insurance company will cover any of their medical care.

- **Coinsurance** is the total percentage an insurance company will pay for a patient's medical care. If a patient has an insurance policy with an 80% coinsurance, that means the insurance company will pay 80% of the cost of the care regardless of the total amount; the remaining 20% will be the responsibility of the patient.

Patients may have private insurance through an employer or through a plan purchased on the **health insurance marketplace** (also called the **exchange**). These private plans are generally one of three main types of MCOs:

- preferred provider organization

- exclusive provider organization

- health maintenance organization

In a **preferred provider organization (PPO)**, providers contract with the insurance company to create a network. If the plan member sees medical professionals included in this network, the member receives the PPO's negotiated rate, which is usually substantially lower than the cash rate. The insurer will then cover some portion of the cost (depending on the plan), and the member pays the specified coinsurance.

PPO plans usually allow members to go directly to a specialist without a referral. Patients may also use out-of-network providers, but the cost covered by the patient will be higher. In addition, the insurance company might not pay for a service a provider requests if the service is not deemed medically necessary.

An **exclusive provider organization (EPO)** is set up the same way as a PPO. The only difference is that patients cannot see out-of-network providers.

A **health maintenance organization (HMO)** requires the member to have a primary care physician who coordinates all care. These physicians are often referred to as **gatekeepers** because their referrals are needed for all

> **Helpful Hint**:
>
> A **pre-authorization** is often necessary for specific medical procedures or services, meaning the insurance company has to approve those procedures/services before they are provided. Without pre-authorization, the patient may be responsible for the full cost of the procedure or service.

services, including specialist visits, diagnostic tests, and medical devices. HMOs only pay for in-network services.

Patients may also have health insurance through public benefits programs:

- **Medicaid** and the **Children's Health Insurance Program (CHIP)** provide health insurance for children, older adults, and people who are disabled or pregnant.

- **Medicare** is a public benefits program that provides health insurance for people ages 65 and older and people with specific disabilities.

- **TRICARE** is a health care program for military personnel, including active-duty US armed forces, those in the National Guard or military reserve, and military family members.

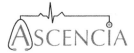

Practice Questions

21. What is a co-pay?

22. What is a deductible?

23. What restrictions are placed on patients with HMO insurance plans?

Financial Barriers to Care

Diabetes care can be very expensive and include some of the following costs:

- visits to endocrinologists and other specialists

- medications, including insulin, antidiabetic agents, and medications for hypertension and hyperlipidemia

- equipment such as BG monitors and insulin pumps

- supplies for monitors, pumps, and insulin injection (e.g., test strips, syringes)

> **Helpful Hint**:
>
> People in the US with type 1 diabetes spend an average of $2,500 a year out of pocket on diabetes care, with the largest expense being testing and injection supplies. About 25% of PWD report rationing insulin for financial reasons.

Insurance coverage for these services and supplies depends on the patient's individual insurance plan. Specialists who work with PWD should be prepared to collaborate with insurance companies to find care options that are affordable to the patient (e.g., therapeutic substitutions for drugs and specific monitoring equipment covered by the insurance plan).

Patients whose insurance will not cover the cost of supplies and patients without insurance will face significant financial barriers to diabetes care. Specialists should be prepared to direct patients toward resources to help cover the costs associated with diabetes care:

- **Patient assistance programs** can provide low-cost medications and supplies to PWD. These are often run by pharmaceutical companies or equipment manufacturers, but they can also be funded by nonprofits or government agencies.

- **Coupon programs,** such as GoodRx, can help lower the cost of medications.

- **Community-funded health care programs** may help patients access supplies for diabetes care.

- **Samples** from medical offices can help patients cover gaps in access to drugs or equipment.

Practice Questions

24. What is a patient assistance program?

25. A specialist learns that a patient is not taking blood pressure medication because it is unaffordable. How can the specialist help this patient?

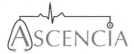

Employment

PWD are protected under the **Americans with Disabilities Act**. The law requires employers to provide reasonable accommodations for PWD to meet diabetes-related needs. These accommodations are typically at no cost to employees and create little to no disruption to the work environment or workflow. To the extent that it does not impede the individual's abilities to perform the core job responsibilities, employers must allow employees to do the following:

- monitor their blood glucose, administer insulin, and consume food or drink to increase BG

- leave for doctor's appointments

- store their insulin in a temperature-controlled environment (if work exposes them to extreme temperatures)

The Americans with Disabilities Act makes it illegal to inquire about an individual's health status or their prognosis before hiring that person; however, it is legal to require a medical assessment as a condition of employment in cases where diabetes care management may impede job performance, productivity, or safety (e.g., if an employee who would be working with heavy machinery might be at risk of experiencing sudden hypoglycemia). These assessments should be based only on the scope of the person's diabetes care and how it relates to work performance capabilities.

> **Helpful Hint**:
>
> Whenever possible, workplaces should provide a private place for employees with diabetes to monitor and manage their glucose levels.

In rare cases, some diabetes-related medical needs may significantly impede the ability to successfully complete core job tasks. Health risks—usually hypoglycemia—may also pose a **direct threat** to workplace safety. PWD can only be fired or denied work if the safety risk cannot be mitigated by reasonable accommodations.

If individuals are being denied opportunities because of their disability statuses (e.g., being denied job opportunities or accommodations that they need to perform their jobs), it is considered **discrimination**. While discrimination against PWD is illegal, it does still occur. Specialists should ensure that patients are aware of their rights so that they can advocate for themselves. The following are some general guidelines for managing accommodations:

- PWD must ask for accommodations at work—the employer has no responsibility to provide accommodations unless specifically requested.

- Employees should document any denial of accommodation or discrimination they experience to help support legal proceedings if needed.

- Health care providers should provide documentation to patients to help them request accommodations.

- Employers are not allowed to access an employee's medical records or communicate with their health care providers without the employee's consent.

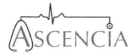

Practice Questions

26. What are the most common workplace accommodations PWD may need?

27. When is an employer permitted to require a medical assessment of an employee?

Chapter 10 Answer Key

1. The two main goals of a management plan are to delay or prevent complications and to improve quality of life.

2. After a care plan is implemented, the health care team should monitor the patient and provide support.

3. The kaleidoscope model of care is based on specific factors and designed in such a way as to allow specialists to tailor an individual's plan for care. As a result, the model is dynamic and can adapt to the needed range of care.

4. The specialist should recommend that the parent use rapid-acting insulin after meals/ snacks instead of preprandial insulin so that the dose can be adjusted for the amount of food consumed.

5. The patient is likely restricting insulin for weight loss.

6. The hormonal fluctuations that accompany puberty lead to insulin resistance, which necessitates adjustments to insulin dosages.

7. The A1C target for most pediatric patients with diabetes is <7%.

8. The honeymoon period of type 1 diabetes is a brief period of remission in which the pancreas produces enough endogenous insulin to maintain normal blood glucose levels.

9. Pediatric patients with type 1 diabetes (T1D) should be screened annually for nephropathy.

10. The target A1C goal for a 67-year-old patient who lives independently and does not have any coexisting chronic conditions or functional or social concerns is 7.0% – 7.5%.

11. Drugs that increase the risk of hypoglycemia, including sulfonylureas, should be used cautiously in older patients.

12. Older patients have a lower fluid volume, which puts them at a higher risk of dehydration.

13. People who have had a kidney transplant typically take high-dose immunosuppressants, which can cause hyperglycemia; as a result, insulin therapy is usually needed to manage hyperglycemia.

14. Lisinopril (an ACE inhibitor) and atorvastatin (a statin) should both be discontinued before pregnancy. Chlorothiazide is a diuretic that may be continued during pregnancy if needed.

15. The current recommendation is to switch to insulin as the first-line therapy during pregnancy.

16. The fasting glucose target range for people with type 1 diabetes who are pregnant is 70 – 95 mg/dL.

17. Insulin needs drop during the first trimester of pregnancy.

18. The patient's insulin needs will drop dramatically immediately after delivery.

19. Used needles should be discarded in a properly labeled sharps disposal container.

20. Patients with type 1 diabetes (T1D) should always check their blood glucose (BG) levels before driving.

21. Co-pays are set payments made by patients every time they seek medical care.

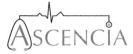

22. A deductible is a set amount that patients must pay before the insurance company will cover any of their medical care.

23. Patients with health maintenance organization (HMO) plans must see in-network providers in order for their insurance to cover the cost, and they must get referrals from their primary care physicians in order to see a specialist.

24. Patient assistance programs provide low-cost medications and supplies. They are usually run by pharmaceutical companies or equipment manufacturers.

25. The specialist can direct this patient-to-patient assistance programs, drug coupons, a cheaper therapeutic equivalent, or drug samples.

26. Most employees with diabetes will require opportunities to monitor their insulin and blood glucose levels, administer insulin, and consume food or drink.

27. An employer can require a medical assessment as a condition of employment, or if diabetes-related issues are interfering with work performance or safety.

Chapter 11 – Standards and Their Applications

The National Diabetes Prevention Program Standards (National DPP)

Current National Standards for Diabetes Self-Management

Diabetes Self-Management Education and Support (DSMES) services must meet certain thresholds regarding their quality in order to be qualify for reimbursement by insurance providers, including Medicare. The quality of a DSMES program is determined by whether it meets various standards created by the American Diabetes Association (ADA) and the Association of Diabetes Care and Education Specialists (ADCES). These standards—updated for 2024—are discussed in the following paragraphs.

Standard 1: The Diabetes Self-Management Education and Support (DSMES) team must look for support, in leadership capacities within the health care community, to help drive both the implementation and sustainability of DSMES.

Standard 2: The DSMES team must understand and identify the target population's demographics, which include race, ethnic/cultural background, and education level. The DSMES team should be culturally sensitive and responsive to an individual's needs, values, and preferences. Equitable DSMES services must include social determinants of health for specific populations to facilitate proper design and delivery. DSMES services must identify and address population barriers that can exist at the health system, payer, health care professional, and individual levels. DSMES services should consider offering telehealth and/or digital interventions to address barrier access and overall satisfaction.

Standard 3: The DSMES team should uphold national standards and implement DSMES services that include evidence-based service delivery, design, evaluation, and quality improvement. The DSMES team, which consists of health care professionals knowledgeable in diabetes, should promote skills acquisition in order to help implement a treatment plan, medical nutritional therapy, or when complicating medical, physical, and psychosocial factors develop.

Standard 4: The DSMES team must use a curriculum that models evidence-based content and delivery. Education regarding novel strategies/advances and support should be documented and shared with other members of the care team.

Standard 5: The DSMES team must be person-centered over the lifespans of the patients with diabetes and based on the needs and priorities of those individuals. The plan encourages all PWD to participate in DSMES in order to facilitate self-care behaviors, problem-solve, make informed decisions, and collaborate with the health care team.

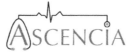

Standard 6: DSMES services should have continuing quality improvement (CQI) techniques to measure their impacts. A systematic evaluation of the outcome and process data is needed to determine areas for optimization and improvement that can result in improved clinical outcomes and reduced costs with reimbursement by third parties.

Practice Question

1. DSMES services will often incorporate continuing quality improvement (CQI) techniques to measure their health impact outcomes. Outcomes may be either "process data" or "outcomes data." Outcome data is considered to be behavioral, clinical, patient-generated (health data), and patient-reported. Healthy eating, healthy coping, and being active would be examples of which type of outcome?

Describing the National DPP Standards

The **National Diabetes Prevention Program (DPP)** is composed of private and public organizations that partner with one another to minimize the risk of type 2 diabetes by providing an evidence-based lifestyle-changing program. The goal of the National DPP is to make it easier for people at risk of developing type 2 diabetes to participate in a high-quality, affordable program.

Partner organizations of the National DPP include state and local health departments, federal agencies, employers, national and community organizations, health care professionals, public and private insurers, businesses that prioritize wellness, and university community education programs. These partner organizations, through the National DPP, have several goals:

- delivering a lifestyle-changing program
- increasing referrals
- increasing participation in lifestyle-changing programs
- ensuring quality and adherence to evidence-based standards
- increasing coverage by public/private insurers and employers
- training community organizations to run the program effectively

The year-long lifestyle-changing programs aim to delay or prevent type 2 diabetes by encouraging participants to eat healthier, improve coping skills, and add physical activities to their daily routines. To enable high-quality partnerships, the organizations must meet specific standards set forth by the CDC in order to achieve specific outcomes. The standards require an approved curriculum, a facilitator (e.g., a lifestyle coach), and a data report to be submitted every 6 months that indicates the impact of the program.

Practice Question

2. The CDC has several requirements for a National DPP lifestyle-changing program; these include an approved curriculum and a lifestyle coach to ensure health changes for the participants. Specifically, the program must last for a specific duration, with a specific number of sessions offered to the participant. In regards to the curriculum, what is the CORRECT delivery time and number of sessions as indicated in the CDC's standard and operating procedures for diabetes prevention?

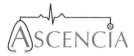

Practice Standards and Guidelines

The practice of diabetes care is guided by multiple professional organizations. These organizations maintain up-to-date, evidence-based practice guidelines that can be referenced by diabetes care and education specialists. The most important of these organizations are briefly discussed below.

The **Association of Diabetes Care and Education Specialists (ADCES)** publishes the **National Standards for Diabetes Self-Management Education and Support (NSDSMES)**, which are updated every five years. These standards provide guidance for the development and maintenance of an effective diabetes education program. They also provide a wealth of resources for diabetes care and education specialists, including a standard curriculum, a library of practice tools, and online courses.

> **Helpful Hint:**
>
> Medicare requires that ADCES- and ADA-accredited diabetes education programs meet the guidelines put forth in the NSDSMES.

The **American Diabetes Association (ADA)** provides diabetes education and resources to both patients and health care professionals. Its patient site (www.diabetes.org) provides educational resources for patients with all types of diabetes. The professional site (https://professional.diabetes.org) houses a wealth of resources for medical professionals, including the **Standards of Medical Care in Diabetes**, a comprehensive set of guidelines for medical professionals caring for patients with diabetes.

The **American Association of Clinical Endocrinology (AACE)** and the **Endocrine Society** also publish clinical practice guidelines that health care providers can reference.

The **Diabetes Prevention Program (DPP)** is a public-private partnership run by the Centers for Disease Control and Prevention with the goal of helping people prevent or delay type 2 diabetes. The program recognizes **lifestyle change programs** that use DPP curricula and materials. These programs provide resources and support so that people can make changes in dietary patterns and exercise. These lifestyle change programs are often covered by insurance and are available to people on Medicare.

The **Diabetes Attitudes, Wishes, and Needs (DAWN) study** is an international survey commissioned by Novo Nordisk (a pharmaceutical company) and the International Diabetes Federation. The study evaluates the psychosocial factors that affect diabetes care and self-management. The results were released in 2001 with the following key findings:

- Self-reported patient adherence to self-management programs was low; providers rated patient self-management behaviors even lower.

- Diabetes-related distress was very common, with a high percentage of patients reporting psychosocial problems but only a small percentage being offered psychosocial care.

- The study identifies common barriers to effective medication therapy, including complicated regimens, patient fatigue, and lack of patient belief in the efficacy of medications.

> **Helpful Hint:**
>
> In the DAWN study, 19% of type 1 patients and 16% of type 2 patients report carrying out all recommended behaviors in their care plans.

- Most patients in the US saw fewer than two medical providers for diabetes care and reported poor communication among care team members.

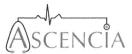

The **DAWN2** study results were released in 2013. This study again emphasizes the psychosocial impact of diabetes diagnosis and care on patients and their families. Key findings include the following:

- There were significant levels of diabetes-related distress among patients and their family members. Non-Hispanic Whites in the US reported higher levels of distress.

- Patients commonly reported feeling discriminated against because of their diabetes diagnosis.

- Most patients want to improve their self-management behaviors but lack access to education and psychosocial resources.

The **Diabetes Control and Complications Trial (DCCT)** is a study published in 1993 on type 1 diabetes. It compares intensive glucose controls (as close to nondiabetic range as possible) with conventional controls that aim only to keep patients asymptomatic. The study, along with follow-up studies over the last 30 years, finds that early, intensive control of glucose levels significantly reduces complications from diabetes.

> **Did You Know**?
>
> The ADCES certifies diabetes care and education specialists, and their guidelines form the framework for the CDCES exam. These resources are available on their website at www.diabeteseducator.org.

Practice Questions

3. Which aspect of diabetes care is examined in the Diabetes Attitudes, Wishes, and Needs (DAWN) study survey?

4. What is the key finding of the Diabetes Control and Complications Trial (DCCT)?

Medical Errors

Medical errors are serious and common problems in health care settings and may be caused by human errors, systemic failures, or both. In some cases, these incidents will cause no adverse effects for the patient; in other cases there could be extensive damage or even fatality. There are many ways to categorize and label medical errors. The following are some of the most common terms:

- A **variance** is a deviation from standard protocols or from a patient's care plan. It may directly impact a patient's care, or it may have no—or only minor—consequences. A patient fall or a medication administered at the wrong time are examples of variances.

- An **adverse event** is a physical injury caused by medical care. It may be the result of substandard care (e.g., incorrect medication administered), or it may be a known risk of care (e.g., hypoglycemia following an initial dose of antidiabetic agent).

- A **sentinel event** is a patient safety event that leads to patient death or serious harm, such as wrong-site surgeries or death by suicide while in care.

- A **near-miss** is an action that could have caused injury to a patient but did not. For example, if a nurse is preparing to administer a medication to the wrong patient but stops after checking the patient's ID bracelet, that is classified as a near-miss.

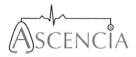

- **Medication errors** are one of the most common medical errors that occur in the United States. Medication errors can occur at any stage: a medication may be incorrectly prescribed, incorrectly dispensed, or incorrectly taken.

- **Polypharmacy**—taking multiple drugs for a single condition—increases the risk of medication errors. Patients taking multiple medications, particularly when prescribed by different clinicians, may be taking medications that amplify or counteract each other. Patients with diabetes who have other chronic health conditions are also at risk for prescription errors (e.g., a patient with congestive heart failure being prescribed a thiazolidinedione).

Patients recently discharged from the hospital are another group at high risk for medication errors. During the hospital stay, health care providers often discontinue, modify, or add medications. When the patient arrives home, they may have both new medications and prior home medications. To prevent medication errors for these patients, medications must be reconciled at discharge and patients should be educated on their new regimen.

The following list includes other common causes of medical errors in diabetes care:

> **Helpful Hint:**
>
> While most facilities now use electronic medical records (EMRs) to help increase team communication and reduce errors, the reconciliation in the system is not always correct.

- incomplete or late laboratory testing

- lack of follow-up with patients

- inadequate or incorrect education on device usage

- focus on diabetes treatment that obscures the need for the treatment of other conditions

No matter how minor a mistake may seem at the time of occurrence, it is important to report it quickly and accurately using the proper channels. The purpose of an **incident report** is to identify the problem that occurred as well as any consequences of the incident. It is not intended to place blame but rather to document the event and track the occurrence of similar events. The documentation should be worded as objectively and honestly as possible because these reports can be used in court if the incident turns into a lawsuit.

Most medical offices—and particularly large settings, like hospitals—will have dedicated reporting systems that operate as part of a larger risk management strategy. **Risk management** is the process of analyzing how these events happen and building processes to prevent them from happening again.

Practice Questions

5. What is a sentinel event?

6. What types of situations put diabetes patients at higher risks for medication errors?

Chapter 11 Answer Key

1. These would be examples of psychosocial and behavioral outcomes.

2. A program that runs at least 1 year with 16 sessions in the first 6 months and 6 sessions scheduled for the last 6 months is correct and based on the 2024 CDC Diabetes Prevention Recognition Program standard and operating procedures. For the organization to have a CDC-recognized curriculum, the National DPP organization must start with an initial 6-month phase, known as the core phase, which requires a minimum of 16 weekly sessions that are offered at least 16 weeks and not more than 26 weeks. Each session is one hour long. The second phase, called core maintenance, is a 6-month phase that requires a minimum of 6 sessions.

3. The Diabetes Attitudes, Wishes, and Needs (DAWN) survey studies the psychosocial factors that affect diabetes care and self-management medical errors.

4. The key finding of the Diabetes Control and Complications Trial (DCCT) is that early, intensive control of glucose levels significantly reduces complications from diabetes.

5. A sentinel event is a patient safety event that leads to patient death or serious harm.

6. Patients with a higher risk for medication errors include those who are taking multiple medications (polypharmacy), patients with other chronic health conditions, and those who have recently been discharged from the hospital.

Chapter 12 – Population Health Strategies and Advocacy

Population Health Strategies

Population health is referred to as the health outcomes of a group of people or individuals that contain the distribution of health outcomes within that group. **Health outcomes** can include morbidity, mortality, and functional status. Diabetes care must be individualized for each person in order to improve population health.

Certified diabetes care and education specialists may work with other professionals or organizations to form a care team and incorporate several ADA standards of care targeted towards a diabetic population. Care teams will often make treatment decisions for PWD that consider **social determinants of health (SDOH)**. SDOH is defined as the environmental, economic, social, and political conditions in which people live, all of which can contribute to health inequalities. The ADA standards in diabetes include several recommendations for diabetes and population health, which include the following:

- Treatment decisions must be timely and made collaboratively with PWD and care partners.

    o These decisions must follow evidence-based guidelines and involve key components with respect to social determinants of health.
    o Treatment decisions must be based on the individual preferences of PWD, financial considerations, and comorbidities.
- The care team should align their approaches with the chronic care model (CCM) for diabetes management.

    o The model requires a person-centered care team with integrated long-term treatment approaches to diabetes.
    o Goal-setting and constant collaborative communication are another component of the model.
    o Elements of the CCM model include delivery system design, self-management support, decision support, clinical information systems, community resources/policies, and quality-oriented culture health systems.
- The care team should incorporate care systems that facilitate in-person and virtual team-based care.

    o Health care professionals who are knowledgeable and experienced in diabetes management should be included.

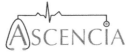

- In order to meet the needs of PWD, the care team should involve patient registries, decision support tools, and support or involvement from the community.
- Care teams should assess the health care maintenance of diabetes by using relevant and reliable data metrics to improve health outcomes and processes.
  - Individuals' goals and preferences must be addressed in addition to the cost of care and patients' burdens to treatment.

Specialists can also play an important role in diabetes prevention for the wider community. Advocacy in the community often focuses on **primary prevention**—interventions that may prevent healthy people from developing diabetes.

Diabetes care and education specialists may participate in community and corporate screening events and health fairs. The goal of these events is to identify people at risk for diabetes and to provide education on eating and exercise habits that can prevent or delay type 2 diabetes. Specialists may also participate in community awareness events through media appearances and/or by posting on social media. The focus of such events is usually to promote awareness of the causes and symptoms of diabetes and to encourage healthy lifestyle changes.

Helpful Hint:

Secondary prevention is the identification of asymptomatic diabetes; **tertiary prevention** is the treatment of disease to prevent its further progression.

Diabetes care and education specialists can also have the responsibility of mentoring and educating other health care staff. They may choose to mentor junior staff or volunteers and may also contribute to continuing education or workplace training activities for providers of other health care specialties. All of these activities should be done within the official structures of the diabetes care and education specialist's workplace.

Practice Question

1. What is primary prevention of diabetes?

Promoting Evidence-Based Care and Education

Due to the increasing costs of diabetes management and rising incident rates, there is a need to broaden strategies that will facilitate improved access to care and outcomes. Improving quality outcomes can alleviate the financial stress and burden of diabetes. Diabetes care and education specialists (DCESs) can aid health care systems with specific delivery models that will improve diabetes care through quality improvement strategies and evidence-based standards.

Specialists are skilled in evidence-based diabetes self-management education and support (DSMES) delivery and include pharmacists, dietitians, and health professionals who have expertise in person-centered care, education, and team collaboration with people with diabetes and their families.

Specialists can deliver broad DSMES that addresses psychosocial, behavioral, clinical, and educational components of care. They can teach PWD and their families how to reduce risks that are associated with diabetes and related conditions. For example, specialists can educate people with diabetes about self-care behaviors that include developing healthy coping skills, being active, eating healthy, taking medication in a timely manner, monitoring, reducing risk, and problem-solving.

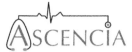

Certified DCESs or (CDCESs) have valuable expertise and knowledge in diabetes care and education; specialists can include clinical psychologists, registered nurses, dietician nutritionists, and physicians, to name a few. Having the **Board Certified-Advanced Diabetes Management (BC-ADM)** credential demonstrates that the specialist has skilled knowledge related to advanced diabetes-related therapeutic skills as well as complex problem-solving and clinical practice skills. Health professionals with a BC-ADM credential are those who have earned a master's degree or higher.

The **Association of Diabetes Care and Education (ADCES)** administers the BC-ADM credential and has a vision of comprehensive care delivery for PWD. The ADCES outlines six areas, or domains, of focus to demonstrate efficiency, effectiveness, and impact on clinical outcomes across diabetes management, care delivery, and education:

1. Clinical Management Practice and Integration
2. Communication and Advocacy
3. Person-Centered Care and Counseling Across the Lifespan
4. Research and Quality Improvement
5. Systems-Based Practice
6. Professional Practice

These areas aim to promote person-centered care with a focus on behavioral health, the use of technology, integration, quadruple aims, and conditions related to diabetes.

Practice Question

2. The CDCES and BC-ADM are both credentials that aim to treat people with diabetes with the goals of improving their health outcomes and decreasing the incidence of diabetes. What are the differences between a board-certified advanced diabetes management (BC-ADM) credential and a person who is a certified diabetes education specialist (CDCES)?

Advocating for People with Diabetes

Specialists will collaborate with various organizations to advance the education, care, and treatment of people with diabetes. For example, specialists may collaborate with the **Diabetes Patient Advocacy Coalition (DPAC)**, an organization comprising PWDs, patient advocates, caregivers, diabetes organizations, health care professionals, and companies. Specialists may even collaborate or become members of the **Association of Diabetes Care and Education Specialists (ADCES)**, which is an organization dedicated to promoting the expertise of the diabetes educator. The ADCES advocates that inpatient teams include diabetes care and education specialists to lead and support quality improvement initiatives for PWDs in hospital settings. The role of a CDCES in a hospital setting is to facilitate change and implement programs to improve outcomes for PWD. Some best practices modeled by CDCES in a hospital or related setting include oversight for person-centered patient and/or family education; oversight in creating educational materials, care coordination, and transitional care support; and best practices for glycemic management as well as technology for continuous glucose monitoring (CGM).

The **Certification Board for Diabetes Care and Education (CBDCE)** oversees the CDCES credential, which authenticates knowledge and expertise in diabetes care and education. Specialists can work or become part of organizations such as DPAC, which support and promote public policy initiatives to improve the

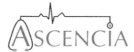

health of PWD. DPAC advocates for safe and quality medications, services, devices, and access to care for people with diabetes. DPAC will advocate at the state and federal levels to improve the access of PWD to health care and affordability. The main issues that the organization will push for are preventive/pre-deductible diabetes coverage, low and predictable costs/rebates, discount pass-through, and individualized treatment choice. DPAC and its affiliates have supported the idea that diabetes coverage should be treated as preventive care in all public and commercial health plans, thereby bypassing any deductibles. Having first-dollar coverage can help PWD afford the health care they need and limit any barriers to diabetes management. Under such circumstances, PWD would also have better access to medical devices, insulin, and other services.

Practice Question

3. Name some of the best practices for a certified diabetes care and education specialist in a hospital setting.

Diabetes Prevention Strategies in At-Risk Individuals

and Populations

In the US, there is a need to focus on primary prevention to address the projected growth of diabetes for at-risk populations. Hispanics, non-Hispanic Black people, and Alaska Natives/American Indians have disproportionately higher rates of diabetes. Both Hispanic and non-Hispanic Black adults with diabetes have higher rates of retinopathy, albuminuria, and poor glycemic control compared to a non-Hispanic White population. Specifically, these minority groups are less likely to get diabetes preventive care, such as retinal examinations, cholesterol screening, and hemoglobin A1c (HbA1c) testing.

Specific models and interventions have been developed to prevent or delay diabetes. For example, the **chronic care model** has been utilized to

- promote partnerships between hospital systems and community groups, and

- integrate the efforts of community health workers to address diabetes for at-risk populations.

Health workers can utilize clinical and population-based strategies to screen, identify, and treat populations with prediabetes. Intervention programs, such as the National Diabetes Prevention Program (DPP), have included interventions such as physical activity, healthy dietary patterns, and weight loss initiatives to prevent or delay diabetes. DPP-type programs have been adapted to include peer support, health educators, and community leaders to improve health outcomes. Programs such as the Fit Body and Soul, a church-based DPP, were developed to prevent diabetes in communities of African descent.

Practice Question

4. How does the chronic care model try to drive care for at-risk populations?

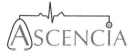

Recognizing the Impact of Disparities

The Centers for Disease Control and Prevention (CDC) highlighted the issue of health disparities and indicated that some ethnic and racial groups are at higher risks of complications such as diabetes. Specialists can help determine which barriers exist that prevent diabetes care and how to improve access to care in both the short and long runs.

As education level and household income decline, the chances of being diagnosed with type 2 diabetes increase. Latino and Hispanic populations, as well as populations of Americans of African descent experience disproportionately higher complications from diabetes. Inaccessibility to healthy food increases disparities among at-risk groups and raises the risk of developing type 2 diabetes. For example, without proper food and nutrition, people will have a more difficult time reaching targeted blood glucose levels and are more susceptible to complications. Interventions to target food insecurity and diabetes include "Food is Medicine" programs (e.g., meals tailored based on medical needs) and federal nutrition assistance programs (e.g., SNAP and WIC).

Due to the burden of diabetes care, which may cause fatigue and exhaustion, addressing health inequities can be challenging for health care teams. Creating health care sector and community partnerships is one way to make more effective use of resources and staffing. Some resources provided by the federal government to support health equity include screening for social determinants of health, skills for addressing challenges and barriers to self-care, referrals to prevention, and enhancing DSMES services.

Practice Question

5. The US Department of Health and Human Services has identified social determinants of health (SDOH) and categorized them into five domains: neighborhood and built environments, health care quality and access, economic stability, education access and quality, and social and community context. Which domain describes an at-risk population that is facing barriers to reliable transportation and access to food?

Collaboration and Diversity, Equity, and Inclusion

The ADCES has created diversity, equity, and inclusion (DEI) practices to deal with racial disparities that impact health and well-being. These practices include the expansion of the level of diversity in leadership and memberships within the ADCES and the creation of several resources geared to train health care professionals to provide culturally appropriate care (e.g., Delivering Culturally Appropriate Care). The ADCES has advocated for equal access through the organization's policies and legislation and has developed a variety of educational programs that address and identify social determinants of health (SDOH) and health equities. Specifically, a DEI council has been established to create a charter and path forward that will focus on reducing disparities in health care based on SDOHs.

Collaboration Within The Health Care Team

Providing the best quality care for patients with diabetes requires a team approach. **Nursing aides**, **medical assistants**, and **patient care technicians** perform a wide range of duties, including taking vital

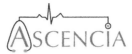

signs, turning the patient in bed, and helping with activities of daily living. Some can also assist with dispensing medications, administering vaccinations, and drawing blood.

The health care team may include some of the following medical professionals:

Helpful Hint:

Nursing aides, medical assistants, and patient care technicians can test capillary blood glucose for patients by using a glucometer.

- **Licensed practical nurse (LPN):** LPNs provide basic nursing care and are required to complete a 12-month nursing program and licensure exam. Depending on the medical facility, LPNs can usually administer oral medications and insulin; they cannot administer intravenous (IV) medications.

- **Registered nurse (RN):** An RN must have an associate degree in nursing or a bachelor of science in nursing. Registered nurses can perform all of the tasks that an LPN does as well as administer all medications, including IV. Registered nurses often oversee LPNs and nursing aides.

- **Nurse practitioner (NP):** An NP has a master's degree in nursing and can examine patients, diagnose and treat diseases, prescribe medications, and (usually) perform procedures. Nurse practitioners can work autonomously under their nursing licenses in the specialties for which they are certified.

- **Physician assistant (PA):** A PA has a master's degree in physician assistant studies and has successfully completed the national board examination. While it varies by state, a PA can usually practice autonomously while maintaining a relationship with a collaborating provider. In general a PA can examine patients, diagnose and treat illnesses, prescribe medications, and perform procedures.

- **Physician (MD or DO):** Physicians have either a doctor of medicine (MD) or doctor of osteopathic medicine (DO) degree. Both are fully trained doctors. A physician can assess, diagnose, and treat patients, prescribe medications, and perform medical procedures.

- **Endocrinologist:** An endocrinologist is an MD who specializes in hormone disorders, such as diabetes. Primary care providers may refer patients to an endocrinologist for advanced management of diabetes.

- **Clinical psychologist:** Clinical psychologists have a doctoral degree but cannot prescribe medications. They diagnose and manage behavioral health disorders with a focus on counseling and therapy.

- **Psychiatrist:** Psychiatrists have a medical degree. They diagnose and manage behavioral health disorders and can prescribe medications.

- **Occupational therapist (OT):** An OT helps patients improve their abilities to perform daily activities. The position requires a master's degree.

- **Physical therapist (PT):** A PT helps patients improve strength and mobility. A PT can diagnose and develop treatment programs and assist with exercise programs. A PT position requires a doctorate.

- **Exercise physiologist (EP):** An EP works with patients to help improve exercise to optimize heart health and body composition. An EP can create a specific exercise program for a patient with diabetes. The position requires a bachelor's degree.

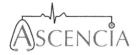

- **Optometrist:** An optometrist holds a doctor of optometry degree. Optometrists examine and prescribe glasses and contact lenses, as necessary.

- **Ophthalmologist:** An ophthalmologist is an MD who specializes in eye care. Ophthalmologists diagnose and provide treatment for eye disorders; they can also perform surgery.

- **Pharmacist:** A pharmacist holds a doctor of pharmacy degree. Pharmacists dispense medications and educate patients about the medications that are prescribed to them by health care providers.

- **Podiatrist:** A podiatrist holds a doctor of podiatric medicine degree and specializes in diagnosing and treating disorders that affect the feet. In caring for patients with diabetes, a podiatrist evaluates the patient's foot and looks for signs of diabetic neuropathy, ulcers or other wounds, and infection.

- **Dietitian/dietitian nutritionist:** Dietitians are credentialed professionals with bachelor's degrees who help patients learn about proper nutrition.

Practice Questions

6. Which of the following health care professionals can prescribe insulin: registered nurse, physician assistant, licensed practical nurse, and/or clinical psychologist?

7. What is a podiatrist's role in diabetic care?

Referrals

A **referral** is generated when a health care provider determines that a patient will benefit from further management or education with a specialist. A referral is ordered by a health care provider and states the person or department that the referral is being sent to as well as the reason(s) for the referral.

When caring for patients with diabetes, referrals are often required for the following issues:

> **Helpful Hint:**
>
> Some insurers require a referral to an in-network specialist or prior authorization of services in order to cover care. The diabetes care and education specialist should work with patients' insurance companies to ensure that the costs of specialist care are covered.

- **Education:** An education referral is made when a patient is newly diagnosed with diabetes or has poor glycemic control. A diabetes care and education specialist helps patients understand how the disease works, what kinds of interventions are available, and how to implement their management plans.

- **Medical nutrition therapy:** Medical nutrition therapy helps provide the patient with recommended foods and meal plans for a dietary pattern that can help prevent complications from diabetes.

- **Exercise:** A referral for exercise can be sent to a physical therapist, exercise physiologist, or an exercise program. Incorporating specific exercises into a patient's daily routine is a large component of managing diabetes.

- **Lifestyle coaching:** A lifestyle coach helps a patient determine personal and other goals and create plans to help achieve those goals.

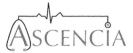

- **Behavioral health:** Diabetes is highly correlated with psychosocial issues, such as depression and anxiety. A psychologist or psychiatrist can evaluate the patient to determine the appropriate diagnosis and treatment.

- **Learning disabilities:** Patients with learning disabilities may have a more difficult time managing their diabetes. Early referral for assistance is key so that they can get the resources necessary to successfully control their diabetes.

- **Medical care:** Patients with diabetes have an increased risk of developing infections and other medical conditions. They should be regularly assessed for complications and referred to the appropriate medical specialist(s) as needed.

- **Medication management:** A referral for medication management can help patients overcome barriers that contribute to the misuse of medication or lack of adherence to a medication regimen.

- **Sleep assessment:** Patients with diabetes are at risk for a number of sleep disorders, including obstructive sleep apnea, restless leg syndrome, and sleep difficulties caused by unstable blood glucose levels. Referral for a sleep study can help diagnose and treat sleep disorders.

- **Financial and social services:** Managing diabetes can be costly. Referrals to social workers for financial and social services can help provide patients with the support they may need to manage their diabetes.

- **Discharge planning and home care:** Discharge planning and home care may include help with medication, patient education, and planning for follow-up appointments. A referral to case management can help ensure that the transition to home is smooth and without errors.

Practice Questions

8. During assessment of a patient recently diagnosed with type 2 diabetes, the nurse notes that the patient cannot identify foods that are high in carbohydrates. Which type of referral would be most helpful for this patient?

9. A patient whose father recently died from complications of diabetes states that she no longer bothers to test her blood glucose because it seems pointless. Which type of referral would be most helpful for this patient?

Chapter 12 Answer Key

1. Primary prevention of diabetes is the implementation of interventions that may prevent healthy people from developing diabetes.

2. People with a BC-ADM credential have more responsibilities concerning complex decision-making. Someone with a BC-ADM credential has the knowledge and competence in advanced diabetes and clinical practice skills that help them make complex decisions, which improves patient outcomes. A person with a BC-ADM credential has the skill set to manage complete patient needs and will help patients with therapeutic problems. Specifically, people with this credential can treat and monitor acute/chronic complications, adjust medications, counsel people with diabetes on lifestyle changes, participate in mentoring/research, and address psychological issues.

3. Some of the best practices for a certified diabetes care and education specialist in a hospital setting include oversight for person-centered patient and/or family education; oversight in creating educational materials, care coordination, and transitional care support; and best practices for glycemic management as well as technology for continuous glucose monitoring (CGM).

4. The chronic care model strives to promote partnerships between hospital systems and community groups as well as integrate the efforts of community health workers to address diabetes for at-risk populations.

5. Built environments are social determinants of health (SDOH) that describe barriers to accessing healthy food, safe spaces for physical activity, and/or reliable transportation to health services. For example, certain groups of people may live in neighborhoods that do not have grocery stores with quality or nutritious food.

6. A physician assistant can prescribe insulin; registered nurses, licensed practical nurses, and/or clinical psychologists cannot.

7. A podiatrist evaluates the feet of patients with diabetes and may look for signs of diabetic neuropathy, ulcers or other wounds, and infection.

8. This patient should be referred to a dietitian for education and medical nutrition therapy.

9. This patient should be referred to a behavioral health specialist, such as a psychologist or psychiatrist.

Practice Test

1. Young children are at high risk for which one of the following complications of hypoglycemia?
   A) pancreatitis
   B) diabetic nephropathy
   C) seizures
   D) cardiac arrythmias

2. A patient who experiences hypoglycemia due to insulin is having which type of adverse drug reaction?
   A) augmented
   B) bizarre
   C) end of use
   D) failure

3. Which of the following complications from diabetes is characterized by damage to the optic nerve?
   A) cataracts
   B) proliferative retinopathy
   C) hypertensive retinopathy
   D) glaucoma

4. A specialist asks a patient to choose a protein bar with the lowest level of sugar based on a list of the first five ingredients. Choosing which one of the following ingredient lists would indicate that the patient needs further education?
   A) whole grain wheat, almond butter, ground chia seeds, cocoa butter, chocolate chips
   B) brown rice protein, dry roasted peanuts, peanut powder, sunflower seeds, honey
   C) dates, walnuts, unsweetened apple, raisins, cinnamon
   D) oats, cane sugar, semi-sweet chocolate chips, cocoa butter, canola oil

5. Which instructions are appropriate for a patient taking Tresiba (insulin degludec)?
   A) Inject dose 15 – 20 minutes before each meal.
   B) Inject dose once daily in either the morning or the evening.
   C) Inhale dose at the start of each meal.
   D) Program insulin pump to deliver a fixed basal infusion.

6. What is the MOST important thing to do if a patient scores high or moderately on the diabetes distress scale (DDS)?
   A) identify healthy coping techniques to practice
   B) refer the patient to a support group
   C) empathize with the patient
   D) refer the patient to a mental health professional

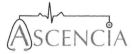

7. A patient with a family history of MODY would like to know about screening for her children. Which type of testing is appropriate?
- A) DNA analysis
- B) plasma glucose levels
- C) A1C
- D) pancreatic antibodies

8. Which of the following measurements would NOT be included in a lipid panel?
- A) LDL-C
- B) serum creatinine
- C) triglycerides
- D) HDL-C

9. What is NOT considered a risk factor for type 1 diabetes?
- A) the presence of pancreatic autoantibodies
- B) exposure to enterovirus during pregnancy
- C) family history of diabetes
- D) gender

10. How does alcohol consumption affect blood glucose levels?
- A) Alcohol has a high sugar content, which causes spikes in glucose levels.
- B) Alcohol causes damage to the pancreas, leading to a reduction in insulin secretion.
- C) Alcohol can mask signs of hyperglycemia.
- D) Alcohol prevents the liver from releasing glucose and causes hypoglycemia.

11. Which diabetes medication should be added to metformin as a second-line treatment in a patient who has atherosclerotic cardiovascular disease (ASCVD)?
- A) GLP-1 receptor agonist
- B) SGLT2 inhibitor
- C) DPP-4 inhibitor
- D) insulin

12. A pediatric health care provider is examining a patient at a health screening fair. Which of the following findings may be indicative of type 1 diabetes and require further investigation?
- A) stomach bloating, swollen lymph nodes, increased thirst
- B) sudden weight loss, blurry vision, muscle weakness
- C) sudden weight gain, ringing in the ears, difficulty sleeping
- D) feeling hungry all the time, increased thirst, waking up at night to urinate

13. Which of the following statements from a patient experiencing recurring hypoglycemic events indicates that further education is required?
- A) "I will make sure to monitor my blood glucose closely and administer insulin based on my glucose values."
- B) "If I do not take my medication as directed, I am at an increased risk of developing diabetes-related complications."
- C) "I should avoid exercise as it can make my blood glucose levels decline rapidly."
- D) "If I feel anxious or shaky, I will check my blood glucose levels immediately."

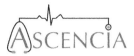

14. Diabetic bullae are MOST likely to appear on which part of the body?
    A) underarms
    B) head
    C) legs, feet, and toes
    D) back

15. A patient with type 1 diabetes has increased her base levels of insulin throughout her third trimester of pregnancy to maintain glucose control. Which of the following statements by the patient indicates she understands how her insulin needs will be affected after she has given birth?
    A) "My insulin dosage will remain the same after delivery."
    B) "I will have to test more frequently because I will require more insulin."
    C) "I should be aware of signs of hypoglycemia because insulin needs will be lowered."
    D) "For the first month after delivery, I may not require insulin."

16. Which type 2 diabetes medication is contraindicated in a patient with NYHA class III heart failure?
    A) Invokana (canagliflozin)
    B) Jardiance (empagliflozin)
    C) Steglatro (ertugliflozin)
    D) Actos (pioglitazone)

17. An adult patient with type 2 diabetes is being monitored for progression of chronic kidney disease. The patient's most recent labs show a GFR of 16. Which of the following symptoms is the patient MOST likely to have?
    A) dehydration
    B) hypokalemia
    C) abdominal pain
    D) peripheral edema

18. Which of the following is a reasonable goal to set for a patient with type 2 diabetes and a BMI of 42?
    A) losing 3% – 5% body weight
    B) maintaining weight between 200 and 220 lbs.
    C) a BMI of 25
    D) losing weight until the patient begins to feel better

19. Under which circumstances might a hiring manager legally be within the right to fire or deny work to an employee with diabetes?
    A) The employee requires intermittent breaks, which can be covered by a coworker, to consume food.
    B) The employee uses paid sick leave to go to monthly doctor's appointments.
    C) The employee must drive during work hours and has a history of severe hypoglycemic episodes.
    D) The employee requires access to the manager's fridge to store insulin.

20. What is the fasting blood glucose target for patients with diabetes who are between six and twelve years of age?
    A) 90 – 150 mg/dL
    B) <80 mg/dL
    C) 120 – 180 mg/dL
    D) 110 – 200 mg/dL

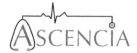

21. Which type of insulin is used by people with diabetes to manage the additional glucose load associated with mealtime?
   A) basal
   B) bolus
   C) endogenous
   D) ultra-long acting

22. A 23-year-old who has never been diagnosed with diabetes is 8 weeks pregnant. She recently had an FBG result of 135 mg/dL. How should the specialist interpret this result?
   A) This result is normal and expected during the first trimester.
   B) The patient has developed gestational diabetes.
   C) The patient has preexisting type 1 or 2 diabetes.
   D) The patient likely did not follow the guidelines for fasting.

23. A patient newly diagnosed with diabetes says that he does not participate in sports and outdoor activities like he used to because he does not sleep well and is always too tired. The specialist should do which one of the following?
   A) make a referral for a sleep study
   B) encourage the patient to exercise even when tired
   C) call the patient's health care provider to request a pharmaceutical sleep aid
   D) explore reasons why the patient is not sleeping well

24. Which class of medications has a black box warning against abruptly stopping the medication?
   A) beta blockers
   B) diuretics
   C) ACE inhibitors
   D) calcium channel blockers

25. Which one of the following is the BEST assessment for cognitive functioning in patients with diabetes?
   A) Mini-Cog
   B) GPCOG
   C) IQCODE
   D) MoCA

26. A patient with a history of nonproliferative retinopathy reports a sudden change in eyesight and flashes of light in one eye. Which one of the following actions is the specialist MOST likely to recommend?
   A) make an appointment with an ophthalmologist as soon as possible
   B) use ophthalmic corticosteroids
   C) seek immediate emergency medical care
   D) place an ice pack over the affected eye to reduce swelling

27. What should be the focus of the first session of a DSMES for the parents of a child who has been newly diagnosed with type 1 diabetes?
   A) how diabetes will progress through the child's life
   B) integrating lifestyle modifications into the child's normal routine
   C) determining activities the child will no longer be able to participate in
   D) providing counselling and education to the parents

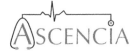

28. Which pharmacokinetic parameters BEST describe Humalog (insulin lispro injection)?
   A)   slow onset, longer duration of action
   B)   slow onset, shorter duration of action
   C)   quick onset, longer duration of action
   D)   quick onset, shorter duration of action

29. After their initial lipid panel, how often should patients with diabetes and no additional risk factors have their lipid levels checked?
   A)   yearly
   B)   every 2 years
   C)   every 4 years
   D)   every 10 years

30. A patient with diabetes is planning to take a business trip next month that involves a long plane ride, and he wants to know how to avoid a DVT. What should the specialist advise?
   A)   Assure the patient that the risk of developing a DVT after a flight is low.
   B)   Advise the patient to take an aspirin before the trip to prevent hypercoagulability.
   C)   Advise the patient to stay hydrated and move around when he is able.
   D)   Suggest that the patient cancel the trip because he is at high risk of getting a DVT.

31. Which one of the following people is MOST at risk for cognitive dysfunction caused by hypoglycemia?
   A)   a pregnant patient with gestational diabetes
   B)   a 3-year-old patient with type 1 diabetes
   C)   a 65-year-old patient who has had type 2 diabetes for 15 years
   D)   a patient with an A1C of 10%

32. A patient who is beginning metformin therapy should be made aware of which potential vitamin or mineral deficiency?
   A)   iron
   B)   calcium
   C)   vitamin B12
   D)   vitamin K

33. The specialist is teaching the parents of a 3-year-old the best way to administer insulin. Which one of the following special considerations should be used when delivering sub-q insulin?
   A)   Keep the same injection site so that it only hurts in one spot.
   B)   Use short, thin needles.
   C)   Insulin should be administered preprandial so that it does not matter how much the child eats.
   D)   Allow pediatric patients to play with supplies for diabetes so they can get used to them.

34. A 67-year-old patient with diabetes was diagnosed earlier in the week with a lower extremity DVT. During a follow-up visit, she reports shortness of breath and chest pain when inhaling and exhaling. Which condition should the health care provider suspect?
   A)   pulmonary embolism
   B)   panic attack
   C)   myocardial infarction
   D)   cerebrovascular accident

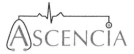

35. Which one of the following is an unmodifiable factor for a 62-year-old patient who is being assessed for type 2 diabetes?
    A) The patient's blood pressure is 189/72.
    B) The patient says her job is very hectic and she rarely sees her family, except on weekends.
    C) The patient has a BMI of 42.
    D) The patient's mother has type 2 diabetes.

36. Which clinical characteristic does NOT need to be considered when selecting a second-line medication to add to metformin therapy?
    A) atherosclerotic cardiovascular disease (ASCVD)
    B) heart failure
    C) chronic kidney disease
    D) chronic obstructive pulmonary disease (COPD)

37. An older adult patient with type 1 diabetes has decreased mobility and a BMI of 17. For which condition is this patient at the MOST increased risk ?
    A) falls
    B) electrolyte imbalance
    C) acanthosis nigricans
    D) pressure ulcer

38. A specialist is meeting with an adult patient who appears disheveled, with her shirt on backwards. The patient's affect is flat, and she responds to questions with one-word answers. The patient usually presents as professional, cleanly dressed, and cheerful. Which one of the following is the BEST question for the specialist to ask?
    A) "You look like you aren't taking care of yourself. Are you having financial difficulties?"
    B) "I am concerned about your appearance. Do you want me to call your family?"
    C) "Please tell me your name, date of birth, and what day it is today."
    D) "Are you having feelings of hurting yourself?"

39. A patient with type 1 diabetes requires frequent adjustments to mealtime insulin doses. Which one of these insulin types is MOST appropriate?
    A) Apidra (insulin glulisine injection)
    B) Lantus (insulin glargine)
    C) Levemir (insulin detemir)
    D) Tresiba (insulin degludec)

40. The parents of a 5-year-old are controlling his type 1 diabetes through a dietary pattern and postprandial insulin administration. Which type of insulin should be used with this regimen?
    A) basal insulin
    B) mixed insulin
    C) intermediate acting
    D) rapid acting

41. What is the primary goal for early medical management of diabetic retinopathy?
    A) relieving pain
    B) slowing disease progression
    C) preventing blurred vision
    D) reversing damage

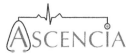

42. What does the DASH diet focus on improving?
   A) blood glucose levels
   B) weight reduction
   C) blood pressure
   D) cholesterol levels

43. A patient is undergoing a procedure that utilizes radiopaque contrast dye. How long before the test should the patient stop taking metformin?
   A) 1 hour
   B) 12 hours
   C) 24 hours
   D) 48 – 72 hours

44. Which one of the following hormones is released if glucagon and epinephrine do not raise blood glucose levels?
   A) cortisol
   B) parathyroid hormone
   C) thyroxine
   D) ghrelin

45. When assessing a patient with poorly controlled diabetes, the health care provider notes that the patient has a quarter-sized wound on the ball of the right foot. A referral to which one of the following specialists is MOST appropriate for this patient?
   A) ophthalmologist
   B) occupational therapist
   C) podiatrist
   D) endocrinologist

46. A 48-year-old man with diabetes is return demonstrating the use of a glucometer with a health care provider. The blood glucose result is 50 mg/dL; however, the patient says he feels fine. What action should be taken?
   A) The patient should ingest 15 grams of carbohydrates.
   B) The health care provider should start an IV and administer IV glucose.
   C) The patient should recheck his blood glucose if symptoms begin to show.
   D) The patient should give himself glucagon with an autoinjector.

47. Which one of the following is recommended for an adult patient with diabetes and risk factors for cardiovascular disease?
   A) Medication is not warranted.
   B) atorvastatin 80 mg
   C) rosuvastatin 40 mg
   D) lovastatin 40 mg

48. A patient with type 1 diabetes says he recently lost his job and health insurance and needs access to insulin and other medically necessary items. What is the BEST action to recommend to the patient?
   A) to immediately find a new job that offers health insurance
   B) to move to a state with expanded Medicaid to ensure health coverage
   C) to sign up for private, subsidized insurance on the health care exchange
   D) to seek out a free clinic in the patient's area for insulin and supplies

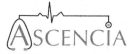

49. How many minutes of moderate aerobic training does the ACSM advise that most people should do per week?
    A) 75 minutes
    B) 60 minutes
    C) 150 minutes
    D) 30 minutes

50. Which OTC medication or supplement can lead to hypoglycemia in patients?
    A) aspirin
    B) pseudoephedrine
    C) niacin
    D) phenylephrine

51. A patient was given 6 units of Humalog (insulin lispro injection) sub-q at 8:30 a.m. At what time should the patient be reassessed and checked for a possible hypoglycemic reaction?
    A) 8:45 a.m.
    B) 9:30 a.m.
    C) 11:30 a.m.
    D) 12:00 p.m.

52. A patient would like to learn to manage his diabetes so that he has more energy and can join his friends on walks. Which type of motivation is this?
    A) intrinsic motivation
    B) self-fulfilling motivation
    C) extrinsic motivation
    D) behavioral motivation

53. A decreased risk of cardiovascular disease is seen in women with which target level of high-density lipoprotein cholesterol (HDL-C)?
    A) 0 mg/dL
    B) 10 – 20 mg/dL
    C) 30 – 40 mg/dL
    D) 50 – 60 mg/dL

54. Defects in which of the following autosomal dominant genes are responsible for MODY?
    A) HNF4A
    B) CEL
    C) IPF1
    D) RFX6

55. The honeymoon period for type 1 diabetes occurs when
    A) a child accepts the disease and is able to participate in care.
    B) insulin is administered at bedtime and causes drowsiness.
    C) a child does not initially require insulin due to sufficient endogenous insulin release.
    D) beta cell function loss requires increasing doses of insulin.

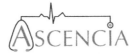

56. In which blood pressure category is a patient with BP readings of 117/79, 112/70, and 115/74?
   A) normal
   B) stage 1
   C) stage 2
   D) hypertensive crisis

57. What is the BEST way to ensure that a patient with diabetes understands how to count carbohydrates after a teaching session about dietary patterns?
   A) assess the patient's comfort level with counting carbs at the next appointment
   B) have the patient calculate the number of carbs in a variety of foods
   C) ask if the patient is comfortable with making these calculations
   D) administer a standardized math test to ensure the patient is able to do simple calculations

58. Which insulin is contraindicated in patients with COPD?
   A) Afrezza (insulin human)
   B) Apidra (insulin glulisine injection)
   C) Basaglar (insulin glargine)
   D) Tresiba (insulin degludec)

59. Which of the following is the BEST public health insurance plan for a new patient with diabetes whose parent is a member of the National Guard?
   A) Medicaid
   B) CHIP
   C) Medicare
   D) TRICARE

60. Why are ketone levels NOT raised in people with HHS?
   A) Hyperglycemia does not reach high enough levels to cause ketoacidosis.
   B) Endogenous insulin production prevents ketoacidosis from occurring.
   C) The slow development of HHS allows the kidneys to remove ketones as they are produced.
   D) Dilutions caused by hypervolemia lower ketone levels.

61. A patient with type 1 diabetes has been newly diagnosed with stage 1 hypertension. Which practice should be recommended by the specialist?
   A) eating a high protein diet
   B) limiting daily fluid intake
   C) monitoring high blood pressure at home
   D) decreasing physical activity

62. A patient being evaluated for diabetes has been instructed to have a fasting blood glucose draw. What is the minimum amount of time after the last meal and drink that this lab can be drawn?
   A) 1 hour
   B) 6 hours
   C) 8 hours
   D) 10 hours

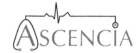

63. Which of the following foods should the specialist recommend to a patient who wants to increase the amount of fiber she eats?
    A) $\frac{1}{2}$ cup of pretzels

    B) 1 apple

    C) 1 cup of lettuce

    D) $\frac{1}{2}$ cup of apple sauce

64. Sodium-glucose cotransporter-2 (SGLT2) inhibitors show evidence for reducing which disease?
    A) hyperlipidemia
    B) heart failure
    C) gastroparesis
    D) pancreatitis

65. A person with type 2 diabetes has severe periodontal disease that causes pain while eating; as a result, he relies on meal replacement shakes. What advice should the nutritionist give this patient?
    A) Liquid foods are more likely to cause hyperglycemia due to high sugar levels.
    B) Eating less may lead to episodes of severe hypoglycemia.
    C) Hypoglycemia is common when people rely on protein shakes and smoothies.
    D) Patients who cannot eat solid foods will require enteral nutrition.

66. At what age do children with diabetes typically begin managing interactions with their care team?
    A) 5 – 11 years old
    B) 14 – 18 years old
    C) 11 – 14 years old
    D) >18 years old

67. If a patient injects 0.15 mL of insulin with an insulin pen that contains a concentration of 100 units/mL, how many units of insulin does the patient receive?
    A) 1 unit
    B) 1.5 units
    C) 10 units
    D) 15 units

68. Which one of the following is an employer legally allowed to do when an employee requests accommodations for diabetes?
    A) access the employee's medical records
    B) ask the employee about unrelated medical conditions
    C) require a medical exam
    D) terminate the employee

69. Which medication for type 2 diabetes could cause patients to experience more frequent yeast infections?
    A) Invokana (canagliflozin)
    B) metformin
    C) Actos (pioglitazone)
    D) glyburide

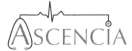

70. A 46-year-old patient with diabetes sees his health care provider for excessive daytime tiredness. The patient also says he has a sore throat and sometimes wakes up gasping for air. What other factor would increase this patient's probability of having sleep apnea?
    A) BMI >45
    B) dawn phenomenon
    C) diabetic peripheral neuropathy
    D) hypertension

71. The parents of a four-year-old are having difficulty managing the child's blood glucose because the child is a picky eater. What advice should the specialist give the parents regarding insulin administration?
    A) "Give a dose in the morning to last throughout the day."
    B) "Administer insulin preprandial so there is coverage before eating."
    C) "Give insulin at bedtime only."
    D) "Adjust insulin dosages based on the amount of food eaten."

72. When should adult patients with diabetes have their first lipid panel done?
    A) immediately after diagnosis
    B) at their one year follow-up appointment
    C) at the age of 40
    D) at the age of 60

73. An adult patient with type 2 diabetes controlled with metformin for the past three years is discussing her recent A1C result of 10%. She says she has been eating a healthy diet and her weight is unchanged. Which one of the following should the specialist anticipate will change in the patient's care plan?
    A) increasing current dosage of medication
    B) lowering carbohydrate intake
    C) increasing exercise
    D) adding a dose of basal insulin

74. The National DPP partners with several organizations to provide PWD access to affordable lifestyle-changing programs, which have been shown to reduce the risk of type 2 diabetes by 58%. In addition to providing lifestyle-changing programs, the National DPP partners with organizations that work to achieve which one of the following goals?
    A) creating a CDC-recognized curriculum for diabetes care and education specialists
    B) training community groups to run an effective program
    C) providing training to community groups on how to screen patients that are at risk of type I diabetes
    D) ensuring that all PWD have access to working technologies

75. A patient newly diagnosed with gestational diabetes has started to check blood sugars each morning. Which fasting value would indicate that the patient is meeting the goal for diabetic control?
    A) 120 mg/dL
    B) 140 mg/dL
    C) 80 mg/dL
    D) 40 mg/dL

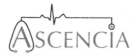

76. The target level for total cholesterol should be less than which number?
   A) 50 mg/dL
   B) 100 mg/dL
   C) 150 mg/dL
   D) 200 mg/dL

77. Amylin affects hunger by doing which one of the following?
   A) stimulating the breakdown of glycogen to raise blood glucose levels
   B) regulating the production of insulin and glucagon
   C) increasing levels of glycogen in the liver
   D) slowing gastric emptying and regulating glucagon release

78. Which OTC medication or supplement can raise blood glucose levels by blocking insulin secretion?
   A) ibuprofen
   B) aspirin
   C) garlic
   D) pseudoephedrine

79. Which feature is used to diagnose the progression of retinopathy to proliferative retinopathy?
   A) microaneurysms
   B) macular edema and decreased visual acuity
   C) abnormal blood vessel growth
   D) exudate in the retina

80. Which of the following foods has the lowest glycemic value?
   A) $\frac{1}{4}$ cup of almonds

   B) 1 slice of whole wheat bread

   C) 1 banana

   D) $\frac{1}{2}$ cup of brown rice

81. Which injection site provides the fastest absorption of insulin?
   A) abdomen
   B) back of the upper arms
   C) buttocks
   D) thighs

82. Which one of the following treatments is appropriate to prevent atherosclerosis in a patient with diabetes who is unable to tolerate statins?
   A) fibrates
   B) ARBs
   C) increased protein in dietary pattern
   D) low carbohydrate, high fat dietary pattern

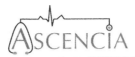

83. What is the purpose of learning the glycemic index system?
    A) to assist people with diabetes in avoiding all foods that contain easily digested sugars
    B) to provide a method to restrict caloric intake
    C) to promote calorie counting to reduce high blood glucose
    D) to enable people with diabetes to easily track their carbohydrate intake

84. Which class of medication can be considered a first-line blood pressure treatment in patients with diabetes?
    A) ACE inhibitor
    B) diuretic
    C) beta blocker
    D) calcium channel blockers

85. A 37-year-old patient with residual cognitive impairments from a recent stroke is participating in a one-on-one class on managing diabetes. The patient has been managing his diabetes since he was first diagnosed in his 20s. Before starting the teaching session, the specialist should assess which one of the following?
    A) the amount of time the patient has available
    B) the patient's ability to perform basic cognitive and physical tasks
    C) whether the patient has a caretaker who is better suited to learn new information and skills
    D) how well the patient has managed diabetes in the past

86. If kidney function is adequate, which medication is a second-line treatment of choice for type 2 diabetes for a patient with chronic kidney disease?
    A) GLP-1 receptor agonist
    B) SGLT2 inhibitor
    C) DPP-4 inhibitor
    D) thiazolidinediones

87. A 58-year-old patient with type 2 diabetes presents to the ED with sweating, nausea, and weakness. She says she had some back pain on and off after working in the garden. Which condition should be ruled out first?
    A) hyperosmolar hyperglycemic state
    B) myocardial infarction
    C) heat stroke
    D) chronic kidney disease

88. A 4-year-old with type 1 diabetes has been in the honeymoon phase for 18 months. What should the specialist tell the parents?
    A) that insulin will soon be required to manage the child's hyperglycemia
    B) that the honeymoon phase will likely last at least another year
    C) that the child will need to go on a low-carbohydrate dietary pattern
    D) that they need to start monitoring the child for hypoglycemic episodes

89. Which medication works by blocking the angiotensin-converting enzyme (ACE)?
    A) lisinopril
    B) amlodipine
    C) furosemide
    D) metoprolol

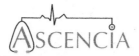

90. Which one of the following is the cause of severe neurological symptoms that can occur during hyperosmolar hyperglycemic state (HHS)?
   A)   hemorrhagic stroke
   B)   decreased glucose transport to brain cells
   C)   seizure activity
   D)   intracerebral dehydration

91. A patient's plan includes the SMART goal of 30 minutes of moderate exercise 5 days per week, a goal the patient says she is unable to meet 75% of the time. Which one of the following actions can the specialist use to support the maintenance stage?
   A)   rewrite the SMART goals so that there is a lower expectation
   B)   start a new plan with a different SMART goal that the patient can 100% achieve
   C)   explore other areas the patient would like to change
   D)   encourage the patient to use a phone app to help track and remind her when to exercise

92. Which one of the following A1C values indicates that a patient who takes oral medication may need to begin insulin therapy?
   A)   2%
   B)   5%
   C)   8%
   D)   11%

93. A patient recently diagnosed with type 2 diabetes says he feels intense fear about potential complications and that this fear is disrupting his self-care. Which treatment is MOST likely to help this patient?
   A)   the use of a continuous blood glucose monitor
   B)   referral to a peer support group
   C)   memory and concentration training
   D)   therapy and anti-anxiety medication

94. Which of the following is a symptom of rhabdomyolysis?
   A)   sweating
   B)   nausea
   C)   muscle pain
   D)   shortness of breath

95. Which condition should be monitored closely in people with diabetes who have been prescribed steroid therapy?
   A)   elevated blood glucose
   B)   elevated blood pressure
   C)   excessive urination
   D)   an increase in heart rate

96. Which one of the following assessments should be done BEFORE a patient is placed on varenicline to help with smoking cessation?
   A)   assess blood pressure
   B)   screen for depression
   C)   recheck A1C
   D)   check pulse

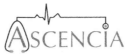

97. What is the target triglyceride level for secondary prevention of cardiovascular disease?
   A) <10 mg/dL
   B) <50 mg/dL
   C) <150 mg/dL
   D) <200 mg/dL

98. A 68-year-old person with diabetes has been treated for cellulitis due to a foot wound. To prevent a future infection, which discharge education is MOST important for this patient?
   A) Take antibiotics until cellulitis is gone.
   B) Check skin on feet daily.
   C) Wear sandals to let feet air out.
   D) Moisturize skin on soles of feet and between toes daily.

99. Which one of the following would NOT lower the glycemic index of a meal?
   A) substituting whole grain pasta for regular pasta
   B) increasing the amount of cream sauce in the dish
   C) adding additional low-starch vegetables to the sauce
   D) having a plain baked potato as a side

100. Which class of medications can reduce overall food intake by regulating appetite?
   A) DPP-4 inhibitors
   B) thiazolidinediones
   C) meglitinides
   D) sulfonylureas

101. Which one of the following patients is exhibiting behaviors that are characteristic of diabulimia?
   A) a patient who is severely restricting calories
   B) a patient who is intentionally vomiting every day
   C) a patient who has musculoskeletal injuries from excessive exercise
   D) a patient who is restricting insulin in order to lose weight

102. Which medical error has occurred in the following scenario:

A patient is waiting for his doctor's appointment when a medical assistant calls the first name and brings the patient to the exam room without verifying the date of birth. The health care provider enters the room and addresses the patient by last name, to which the patient responds that the last name is incorrect.
   A) adverse event
   B) sentinel event
   C) documentation error
   D) near-miss

103. An adult patient with type 2 diabetes has an A1C of 10.2% despite being optimized on oral medications. Which one of these treatments could be recommended by the specialist?
   A) insulin lispro 15 minutes before meals
   B) insulin aspart once daily at bedtime
   C) human insulin NPH 30 minutes before meals
   D) insulin glargine once daily in the evening

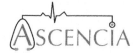

104. Blood test results for a patient being assessed for type 1 diabetes show the presence of pancreatic autoantibodies and fasting blood glucose results at 98 mg/dL. In which stage of type 1 diabetes is the patient?
   A) prediabetes
   B) stage 1
   C) stage 2
   D) stage 3

105. Which one of the following would NOT be included in a 504 plan for a child with diabetes?
   A) requiring trained personnel to assist in the child's care
   B) scheduling for meal and snack breaks
   C) having access to blood sugar testing at any time
   D) providing extra tutoring for learning assistance

106. Which option represents a factor associated with SDOH that can impact the treatment or health outcome of an individual?
   A) the composition of the care team
   B) food insecurity
   C) the knowledge and expression of the care team
   D) individual's preferences for care

107. Which of the following allows glucose to enter cells?
   A) carbohydrates
   B) insulin
   C) triglycerides
   D) hexamers

108. What should a person with diabetes and hyperthyroidism who feels nauseous and dizzy do FIRST?
   A) eat an apple
   B) drink 4 oz of chocolate milk
   C) seek immediate medical care
   D) check blood glucose levels

109. How should a patient be instructed to take the antidiabetic agent Symlin (pramlintide acetate)?
   A) Inject medication subcutaneously immediately prior to meals.
   B) Inhale dose at the beginning of a meal.
   C) Inject medication subcutaneously once weekly.
   D) Take medication 30 minutes before breakfast.

110. A health care provider is providing dietary instructions to a patient with type 2 diabetes and normal kidney function. Which statement by the patient requires intervention by the provider?
   A) "I should limit cholesterol intake to 200 mg/day."
   B) "I should eat a very low carbohydrate dietary pattern."
   C) "My protein intake should be 15% – 20% of my daily calories."
   D) "Fiber will improve my carbohydrate metabolism and lower my cholesterol."

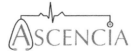

111. Which percentage of insulin administered to a 7-year-old patient with type 1 diabetes is basal?
    A) 70% – 80%
    B) 30% – 40%
    C) 90%
    D) 50% – 60%

112. A patient with diabetes was admitted to the hospital for treatment of sepsis due to an infected foot ulcer. The creatinine is 3.2 mg/dL. Which condition does this value indicate?
    A) myocardial infarction
    B) acute liver failure
    C) osteomyelitis
    D) acute kidney injury

113. A 14-year-old patient with type 2 diabetes is self-managing insulin administration and insists that she has followed a healthy dietary pattern as evidenced by an 8-pound weight loss. Her recent A1C is 7.5%. This patient should be screened for which one of the following?
    A) thyroid disease
    B) celiac disease
    C) eating disorders
    D) depression

114. Which blood pressure medication works by blocking the movement of calcium in vascular muscles?
    A) Norvasc (amlodipine besylate)
    B) Prinivil (lisinopril)
    C) Diovan (valsartan)
    D) Lopressor (metoprolol tartrate)

115. Per ADA guidelines, a person who has previously screened positive for prediabetes should continue to be screened at which frequency?
    A) yearly
    B) every other year
    C) every three years
    D) never

116. A 76-year-old patient with a history of congestive heart failure, hypoglycemic episodes, and a low compliance with medication regimens has developed type 2 diabetes. The specialist has been working unsuccessfully with the patient for several months to control the diabetes through dietary patterns. Which treatment is MOST beneficial for this patient?
    A) sliding scale insulin ACHS
    B) a single dose of long-acting basal insulin
    C) sulfonylurea
    D) implementing a stricter dietary pattern

117. Which of the following BEST describes a correction factor of 30?
    A) Patients must wait 30 minutes before injecting their insulin.
    B) Before the next meal, 30 units of bolus insulin are needed.
    C) One unit of rapid-acting insulin will lower the patient's BG by 30 mg/dL.
    D) Taking 30 units of basal insulin at bedtime will correct for hyperglycemia.

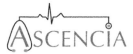

118. A person with diabetes has just eaten four hard candies after experiencing shakiness and dizziness. According to the 15-15 rule for the treatment of hypoglycemia, which one of the following should be the person's next step?
    A) immediately check blood sugar
    B) take 15 grams of glucose gel
    C) check blood glucose in 15 minutes
    D) wait 15 minutes to see if the person is feeling better

119. A patient's continuous glucose monitor (CGM) shows that he has been having hypoglycemic episodes; however, the patient reports that he has not noticed any symptoms of hypoglycemia. Which endocrine process has been disrupted in this patient?
    A) somatostatin, regulating insulin production
    B) amylin, slowing gastric emptying
    C) epinephrine, stimulating the sympathetic nervous system
    D) thyroxine, stimulating metabolic processes

120. What is the blood pressure target for an adult patient with diabetes and a low risk of cardiovascular disease?
    A) <120/80 mm Hg
    B) <130/80 mm Hg
    C) <140/90 mm Hg
    D) <150/90 mm Hg

121. A patient with prediabetes has lost a significant amount of weight through extreme calorie restriction. She currently has a BMI of 19 but has continued her dietary pattern and reports being worried that she is "too fat to be healthy." Which condition should the specialist suspect?
    A) anorexia nervosa
    B) bulimia nervosa
    C) diabulimia
    D) binge eating disorder

122. Which of the following processes is affected by liver failure?
    A) beta cell release of insulin
    B) secretion of glucagon by alpha cells
    C) breakdown of glycogen into glucose
    D) the use and storage of glucose by cells

123. A person with type 1 diabetes is in the ED with fruity breath, dry mouth, tenting skin, and blood glucose of 323 mg/dL. Which lab should be drawn to determine the cause of symptoms?
    A) urinary ketones
    B) potassium
    C) arterial blood gas
    D) hematocrit

124. Eating stimulates the pancreas to release insulin in how many waves?
    A) 1
    B) 2
    C) 3
    D) 4

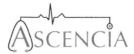

125. A person with diabetic neuropathy reports improvement of symptoms after starting gabapentin and tramadol. Which assessment is MOST important for this person?
   A) neuro
   B) sensory
   C) integumentary
   D) psychosocial

126. What is an immediate outcome goal following an ADCES-approved DSMES program?
   A) the ability to return demonstrate skills taught during class
   B) improved blood pressure
   C) A1C that is decreased by 10%
   D) the patient reporting an improved quality of life

127. Novolin R (insulin human) will exert its maximum effect approximately how many hours after injection?
   A) 0.5 hours
   B) 3 hours
   C) 10 hours
   D) 24 hours

128. A patient with type 1 diabetes feels shaky and nauseated after a morning run. His blood glucose is 62 mg/dL. Which one of the following is the BEST snack to correct his hypoglycemia?
   A) chocolate bar
   B) apple juice
   C) peanut butter sandwich
   D) cottage cheese

129. A patient with type 2 diabetes has had significant weight loss success after bariatric surgery but reports feeling tired lately. What should the specialist assess regarding this patient's nutritional habits?
   A) whether the patient regularly takes vitamin and mineral supplements
   B) whether the patient follows a low-carb dietary pattern
   C) whether the patient consumes a glass of water during each meal
   D) whether the patient eats three meals per day with no snacks in between

130. Which one of the GLP-1 receptor agonists can be administered as a once-weekly injection?
   A) Victoza (liraglutide)
   B) Rybelsus (semaglutide)
   C) Byetta (exenatide)
   D) Trulicity (dulaglutide)

131. A 29-year-old patient being evaluated for type 1 diabetes says she never feels full enough no matter how much she eats. What is the most likely explanation for this phenomenon?
   A) Overeating has caused the patient's appetite to increase.
   B) A lack of insulin is preventing cells from using glucose.
   C) The additional calories consumed by the patient are overstimulating insulin production.
   D) Excess glucose is being excreted through urination.

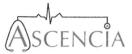

132. How should an A1C goal be set for an older patient with early onset Alzheimer's disease?
   A)   A1C levels should not be used to guide treatment for this patient.
   B)   Use preprandial blood glucose monitoring to estimate A1C.
   C)   Set an A1C target of 6.5% or less.
   D)   Set an A1C target of 8% or less.

133. Which decongestant is recommended for a patient with type 2 diabetes?
   A)   pseudoephedrine
   B)   phenylephrine
   C)   oxymetazoline
   D)   none

134. Which of the following is characteristic of diabetic peripheral neuropathy?
   A)   increased reflexes in ankles
   B)   numbness radiating from the neck down
   C)   sensory loss in stocking-glove distribution
   D)   pain that improves at night

135. Which of the following screenings is NOT required for a pediatric patient with type 1 diabetes?
   A)   celiac disease
   B)   dyslipidemia
   C)   obstructive sleep apnea
   D)   thyroid

136. How many medications are initiated for treatment if a patient's blood pressure levels are >160/90 mm Hg?
   A)   1
   B)   2
   C)   3
   D)   4

137. A person with impaired executive functioning caused by poorly controlled type 2 diabetes would have difficulty with which one of the following?
   A)   performing tasks that require planning and sequencing.
   B)   learning new skills quickly.
   C)   memorizing and paying attention to details
   D)   regulating emotions

138. Which setting is BEST for an event aimed at the primary prevention of diabetes?
   A)   meeting with patients with diabetes in their homes to teach the proper administration of insulin
   B)   a community fair that screens individuals for diabetes risk
   C)   teaching a diabetes support group about dietary patterns and choices
   D)   conducting follow-up calls to improve glycemic control in patients who are newly diagnosed with diabetes

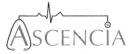

139. Which medication is appropriate for a 65-year-old patient with diabetes and atherosclerosis?
    A) simvastatin 20 mg
    B) pravastatin 40 mg
    C) lovastatin 40 mg
    D) atorvastatin 40 mg

140. A 19-year-old patient reports excessive hunger and thirst, as well as increased frequency of urination. Her FBG result is 200 mg/dL, and no pancreatic autoantibodies are detected in a blood sample. Which type of further testing is expected for this patient?
    A) pancreatic biopsy
    B) genetic testing
    C) urine glucose test
    D) thyroid test

141. What should a patient with type 2 diabetes do before becoming pregnant?
    A) transition from an ACE inhibitor to another blood pressure medication
    B) decrease insulin dosage to prevent hypoglycemia
    C) switch from metformin to a sulfonylurea
    D) take a 75 g OGTT to assess for gestational diabetes

142. Which ingredient in OTC medications or supplements can cause hyperglycemia?
    A) carbohydrates
    B) ginger
    C) alcohol
    D) garlic

143. A 62-year-old patient with diabetic nephropathy has been managing the progression of the disease through a dietary pattern. Which one of the following statements is MOST concerning?
    A) "I take my blood pressure every morning and before taking blood pressure medication."
    B) "I have cut all meat products out of my diet and eat mostly vegetables now."
    C) "My last A1C was 6.4%, down from the previous of 8.3%."
    D) "I am still in stage 3 CKD."

144. The MOST common side effects of metformin affect which system?
    A) cardiovascular
    B) gastrointestinal
    C) neurological
    D) pulmonary

145. Which type of fat is found in flax seed and fatty fish oil?
    A) unsaturated fats
    B) monounsaturated fats
    C) omega-3 fatty acids
    D) trans fatty acids

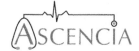

146. Which other hormone is released with insulin to cause a feeling of fullness after eating?
    A) somatostatin
    B) cortisol
    C) pancreatic polypeptide
    D) amylin

147. A patient with A1C and diabetes wants to know what his HgbA1C level of 6.9% means. Which response from the health care provider is MOST appropriate?
    A) "Your level is within target range and indicates good glycemic control."
    B) "Your level is too high, and you will need to increase your medications."
    C) "Your medication has made your blood glucose too low."
    D) "Your primary health care provider may want to place you on an insulin pump."

148. A patient who has watched a video and received education from a health care provider is preparing to self-administer insulin under the provider's guidance. Which one of the following actions by the patient represents learning in the psychomotor domain?
    A) taking notes during the video to refer back to
    B) using de-stressing techniques when feeling overwhelmed by new information
    C) asking questions about how insulin works
    D) setting the correct dose and self-administering insulin with the insulin pen

149. Which one of the following indications would make a 64-year-old patient a good candidate for insulin therapy?
    A) an A1C of 7%
    B) symptoms of hypoglycemia
    C) blood glucose of 220 mg/dL
    D) symptoms of hyperglycemia

150. A 54-year-old patient with diabetes says that she frequently has a very dry mouth despite staying hydrated. Which treatment should the specialist suggest?
    A) Only brush teeth once a day.
    B) Use a xylitol mouthwash.
    C) Increase sodium consumption.
    D) Chew on ice cubes.

151. How many grams of carbohydrates are in a snack of one cup of milk and half a banana?
    A) 30 grams
    B) 20 gram
    C) 100 grams
    D) 45 grams

152. How does glyburide work to lower blood glucose?
    A) It causes the kidneys to excrete more glucose.
    B) It stimulates the pancreas to make and release insulin.
    C) It reduces glucose output from the liver.
    D) It reduces the absorption of glucose.

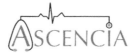

153. A 32-year-old White, non-Hispanic man with a maternal family history of type 2 diabetes is concerned about his risk of developing the disease. Which of the following factors creates the highest risk for this person?
   A)   gender
   B)   family history
   C)   race
   D)   age

154. A specialist is teaching a class on managing diabetes through pregnancy and postpartum with a group of new patients who have been diagnosed with gestational diabetes. Which one of the following is important to teach this group regarding complications from diabetes during the third trimester?
   A)   DKA may develop at lower blood glucose levels.
   B)   Insulin requirements will be lower than at other times during the pregnancy.
   C)   Higher glucose levels will cause slow growth of the fetus.
   D)   The risk for preeclampsia is reduced close to delivery.

155. A 33-year-old patient is using a pen to inject her insulin. At which angle should she be instructed to inject her insulin?
   A)   10 degrees
   B)   30 degrees
   C)   45 degrees
   D)   90 degrees

156. A patient with increasing difficulty managing her diabetes says that she is tired of dealing with it. Which resource should the specialist explore with the patient?
   A)   keeping a dietary pattern diary
   B)   psychosocial care
   C)   budgeting to be able to better afford medications
   D)   implementing home care

157. A 21-year-old male is using a traditional insulin pump with a continuous glucose monitor. How often should he change the infusion set?
   A)   once daily
   B)   every 2 – 3 days
   C)   once weekly
   D)   every 14 days

158. A patient with diabetes who has had bariatric surgery reports that she sometimes develops sudden diarrhea and feels dizzy after eating. Which condition is she MOST likely experiencing?
   A)   gastroparesis
   B)   hypotension
   C)   dumping syndrome
   D)   *Clostridioides difficile* infection

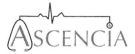

159. Which one of the following insulin injection options is the MOST frequently used method for delivery?
    A) insulin pen
    B) insulin pod
    C) insulin pump
    D) insulin vial and syringe

160. A patient with diabetes has recently lost his job and is struggling to pay for his diabetes care. Since his family relied on his income, he is also receiving a lot of pressure from them to improve their financial situation. The patient would MOST benefit speaking with which care provider?
    A) care manager
    B) social worker
    C) case manager
    D) nurse practitioner

161. A 5-year-old child with diabetes who is toilet trained begins wetting the bed at night. Which action should the specialist suggest?
    A) to discipline the child for this behavior
    B) to check the child's blood sugar before bed
    C) to limit liquids at night to prevent bed wetting
    D) to increase the child's evening meal insulin dose

162. When assessing a new patient, the specialist notes that the patient has been prescribed propylthiouracil. Which condition does this patient likely have?
    A) hypothyroidism
    B) hyperthyroidism
    C) Addison's disease
    D) Cushing's syndrome

163. Which pharmacokinetic parameters BEST describe basal insulin?
    A) slow onset, longer duration of action
    B) slow onset, shorter duration of action
    C) quick onset, longer duration of action
    D) quick onset, shorter duration of action

164. Which instructional strategy is MOST appropriate for a patient who would like more practice with administering insulin and checking blood sugar?
    A) group discussion
    B) lecture
    C) simulation
    D) modeling

165. Which one of the following is a sign of sudomotor dysfunction?
    A) anhidrosis
    B) palpitations
    C) incontinence
    D) moist, peeling skin

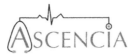

166. A patient with diabetes is enrolled in a DSMES program and has just completed the first session. When should the patient schedule the next follow-up?
    A) 3 – 6 months
    B) one week
    C) 2 – 4 weeks
    D) one year

167. When calculating an insulin-to-carb ratio, approximately how many grams of carbohydrates are covered by one unit of rapid-acting insulin?
    A) 2 – 5 grams
    B) 12 – 15 grams
    C) 25 grams
    D) 50 grams

168. A patient with diabetes is working with a specialist to develop a weight loss plan. The patient was recently diagnosed with cardiovascular autonomic neuropathy (CAN). How might this condition affect his ability to follow a traditional dietary pattern and exercise plan?
    A) Numbness in limbs may limit his ability to move.
    B) He may require higher levels of insulin when exercising.
    C) His sodium-restricted dietary pattern may cause electrolyte imbalances.
    D) He may experience exercise intolerance.

169. Which supplement provides the MOST benefit to a patient with diabetic neuropathy?
    A) chromium
    B) coenzyme Q10
    C) probiotics
    D) garlic

170. A patient with type 2 diabetes, whose A1C has decreased from 7.1% to 6.4% as a result of increased exercise and strict portion control, wants to know if he is still considered diabetic. What is the BEST response by the specialist?
    A) "Your lab values are not showing enough improvement to be considered not diabetic."
    B) "You no longer have to follow a special diet."
    C) "Your A1C is lower, but you need to be stricter with your diet to lower it further."
    D) "How would your lifestyle choices change if you were no longer considered diabetic?"

171. A highly athletic adult patient with type 1 diabetes is having difficulty managing his blood sugar on intense workout days. Which advice should the specialist give to this patient?
    A) to eat a higher carb meal prior to exercise
    B) to hold insulin on those days before exercise
    C) to reduce exercise to half the intensity of normal
    D) to buy an insulin pump to reduce the need to monitor and self-administer insulin when exercising

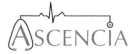

172. An LPN is reviewing orders for a patient and prepares to administer the patient's insulin prior to a meal. The order is for 10 units of regular insulin administered via IV. Which action by the LPN is correct?
    A) administering the regular insulin through the IV
    B) reporting to the RN
    C) holding the dose
    D) administering the same dose subcutaneously

173. A patient with diabetes and a sedentary lifestyle is discussing ways to improve health and increase exercise. Which exercises are LEAST appropriate for this patient to start with?
    A) aerobics that progressively increase
    B) high-intensity interval training
    C) weight training
    D) balance and stability

174. How often should an adult patient who is newly diagnosed with type 2 diabetes have a comprehensive foot exam?
    A) every provider visit
    B) biannually
    C) as needed when there is a wound
    D) annually

175. Fragmentation in health policy and health service delivery in the US has led to persistent inequities and stagnation in diabetes care. As a result, specialists have focused on interprofessional teams, community partnerships, and working with organizations to deliver different levels of care. What is it called when the level of care or vision attempts to improve clinical outcomes across diabetes management and care delivery?
    A) accomplishing quadruple aim
    B) person-centered care strategies
    C) leveraging technology
    D) driving integration

Answer Key

1. C: Children under three years of age are vulnerable to low blood sugar levels. Setting loose blood glucose (BG) targets can prevent hypoglycemic events that can lead to central nervous system damage including seizures, blindness, and cognitive impairment.

2. A: Augmented reactions are predictable reactions arising from the pharmacological effects of the drug. They are typically dependent on dose.

3. D: Increased pressure and swelling in the eye can damage the optic nerve, leading to glaucoma. This damage may result in a loss of vision or complete blindness.

4. D: Per US Food and Drug Administration (FDA) rules, ingredients are listed on a food's nutrition facts label in order of predominance. An ingredient further along the label indicates a lesser amount is used in the food. The protein bar with cane sugar as the second ingredient has the highest level of added sugar; therefore, this choice indicates that the patient needs further education on reading nutrition labels.

5. B: Tresiba (insulin degludec) is an ultra-long-acting insulin that can be injected once daily in either the morning or evening.

6. D: Patients scoring moderately or high on the diabetes distress scale (DDS) would benefit from direct professional mental health support.

7. A: Mature onset of diabetes of the young (MODY) is a group of genetic disorders that causes beta cell dysfunction. Hyperglycemia is present; however, there are no pancreatic antibodies. Genetic testing (DNA analysis) may be used to screen for MODY.

8. B: Serum creatinine, a measure of renal functioning, is not included in a lipid panel.

9. D: Type 1 diabetes affects all genders equally; gender is not a considered a risk factor.

10. D: Since the hepatic system is unable to process alcohol, it prevents the liver from releasing enough glucose for up to 12 hours. Hypoglycemia is a major concern for people with diabetes who drink alcohol, especially at night. The specialist should suggest the patient avoid drinking alcohol on an empty stomach and to have a snack if drinking alcohol prior to bed.

11. A: For patients with ASCVD, a glucagon-like peptide-1 (GLP-1) receptor agonist with proven cardiovascular benefits is recommended.

12. D: Signs of type 1 diabetes include polyphagia (increased hunger), polydipsia (increased thirst), and polyuria (increased urine output). Swollen lymph nodes, muscle weakness, bloating, ringing in the ears, and difficulty sleeping are associated with other medical diagnoses.

13. C: Exercise should be encouraged since it can help regulate blood glucose levels by improving insulin sensitivity. Patients who experience hypoglycemia should be instructed to check blood glucose levels before and after exercise and adjust their dietary patterns and medications accordingly.

14. C: Diabetic bullae most commonly appear as blisters on the lower extremities.

15. C: Immediately after giving birth, the insulin needs of the mother will reduce drastically. During the first few days, frequent testing and a decrease in the insulin dosage will be required. The patient will

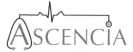

need to be cognizant of hypoglycemic episodes while adjusting to the new insulin doses; however, within the first week, insulin requirements will rise back to the patient's baseline.

16. D: Actos (pioglitazone) is a thiazolidinedione. Thiazolidinediones are contraindicated in patients with New York Heart Association (NYHA) class III and class IV heart failure.

17. D: Glomerular filtration rate (GFR) reflects kidney function. A lower number indicates that the disease is worsening. Since the kidneys are unable to maintain fluid balance, fluid builds up within the body and is reflected by worsening edema. Dialysis is required to prevent pulmonary edema and congestive heart failure.

18. A: Losing 3% – 5% body weight is a reasonable goal that will provide health benefits for the patient.

19. C: It is permitted to fire or deny work to employees with diabetes due to their health condition only in circumstances where the safety risk cannot be mitigated by reasonable accommodations.

20. C: The fasting blood glucose (FBG) target for children between the ages of six and twelve is between 120 and 180.

21. B: Bolus insulin, also called mealtime insulin, is administered by people with diabetes to manage the additional glucose load associated with mealtime.

22. C: Hyperglycemia that presents during the first trimester likely indicates pre-existing type 1 or 2 diabetes. Gestational diabetes does not usually manifest until the second or third trimester.

23. D: The specialist should gather more information on why the patient is not sleeping well. Patients with diabetes are at risk for many sleep disorders, including restless leg syndrome, sleep apnea, and difficulty sleeping as a result of hypo- or hyperglycemia.

24. A: Beta blockers carry a black box warning since abruptly stopping use of this type of medication can cause rebound hypertension, tachycardia, arrythmia, or angina.

25. D: The Montreal Cognitive Assessment (MoCA) is recommended by the American Diabetes Association (ADA) to assess cognitive functioning in patients with diabetes.

26. C: Sudden changes in eyesight and flashes of light suggest a retinal detachment, which is a medical emergency that requires prompt surgical treatment to preserve sight.

27. B: The first session of a diabetes-self management education and support program (DSMES) should be aimed at discussing behavioral health and lifestyle modifications with both the child and family. The focus should not be on excluding previous activities but on making them work while providing management of diabetes.

28. D: Pharmacokinetic parameters define how insulin acts in the body. The rapid-acting insulin Humalog (insulin lispro injection) has a quick onset and shorter duration of action.

29. C: Following an initial lipid panel, patients with diabetes and no additional risk factors should have their lipid levels checked every four years.

30. C: The main factors that increase the risk of deep vein thrombosis (DVT) formation are venous stasis, hypercoagulability, and endothelial damage. Modifiable factors that the patient can control include preventing venous stasis through increased mobility and preventing dehydration that may cause hypercoagulability.

31. B: Very young patients with type 1 diabetes have a higher risk of developing cognitive dysfunction caused by hypoglycemia.

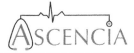

32. C: There is a relationship between long-term metformin use and vitamin B12 deficiency.

33. B: Short, thin needles reduce the probability of pain or discomfort and are therefore most effective in administering subcutaneous (sub-q) insulin.

34. A: A deep vein thrombosis (DVT) that has dislodged may travel toward the lungs and occlude a pulmonary artery, causing a pulmonary embolism.

35. D: An unmodifiable risk factor is one that the patient cannot change, including genetics. The patient is at a higher risk for developing diabetes due to family history.

36. D: Chronic obstructive pulmonary disease (COPD) is not a condition that needs to be considered when selecting a second-line medication to add to metformin therapy.

37. D: A decrease in the hypodermis due to being underweight (BMI <19) puts a patient at risk for developing pressure ulcers over the bony prominences. Due to mobility issues, this person is at a two-fold risk.

38. C: Since the appearance and behavior of the patient have noticeably changed, it is important to first determine the patient's cognitive status. Asking the patient to share her name, date of birth, and what day it is will determine if the patient is alert and oriented. The specialist should then ensure that the patient is safe at home and determine whether she is experiencing depression.

39. A: Apidra (insulin glulisine) is a rapid-acting insulin that controls blood sugar around mealtimes.

40. D: Controlling postprandial hyperglycemia in children is accomplished with rapid-acting insulin. Action onsets within 5 – 15 minutes, peaks in 1 –2 hours, and lasts for approximately four hours.

41. B: Slowing the progression of the disease through tight glycemic control and the treatment of hypertension is the main goal of early medical management.

42. C: The Dietary Approaches to Stop Hypertension (DASH) diet is aimed at reducing blood pressure by focusing on including non-starchy vegetables and whole grains while restricting sodium and saturated fats. While the DASH diet may improve blood glucose levels, weight loss, and cholesterol, it is aimed at controlling hypertension.

43. D: To prevent the possibility of lactic acidosis, metformin should be stopped 48 – 72 hours prior to exposure to radiopaque contrast dye.

44. A: If the body is unable to raise blood glucose levels through the release of glucagon and epinephrine, the body's endocrine system will secrete cortisol and growth hormone to reverse hypoglycemia.

45. C: Podiatrists specialize in treating and managing disorders of the feet and are able to assess the patient.

46. A: A blood glucose level under 54 mg/dL is considered stage 2 hypoglycemia and should always be treated, even if the patient has no obvious symptoms. Since the patient is conscious, oral intake of the standard treatment of 15 grams of carbohydrates is a safe action.

47. D: Since the patient is considered moderate risk, lovastatin 40 mg, a moderate-intensity statin therapy, is recommended.

48. C: Job loss is a qualifying life event that will allow the patient to purchase private health insurance immediately, which will be subsidized based on income.

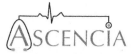

49. C: The American College of Sports Medicine (ACSM) advises that individuals participate in at least 150 minutes of moderate aerobic exercise per week.

50. A: Aspirin has been shown to decrease levels of blood sugar and can lead to hypoglycemia, especially in patients taking sulfonylureas.

51. B: Humalog (insulin lispro injection) is fast-acting insulin, with onset of action beginning 15 minutes after injection. Humalog peaks 30 – 90 minutes after administration, and during this peak time the patient is most likely to experience a hypoglycemic reaction. It would be too early to check the patient at 8:45 a.m., and checking the patient at 11:30 a.m. or later is too late.

52. C: Extrinsic motivation is the incentive to engage in a specific activity in order to gain a reward. In this case, the patient wants to participate in activities that are enjoyable and allow him to be with his friends.

53. D: High levels of high-density lipoprotein cholesterol (HDL-C) are associated with a decreased risk for cardiovascular disease. In women, an HDL-C target level of 50 – 60 mg/dL is ideal.

54. A: The hepatocyte nuclear factor 4 alpha (HNF4A) gene is autosomal dominant, while the other genes listed are recessive. Defects in these genes have been isolated in diagnosing mature onset diabetes of the young (MODY).

55. C: Children diagnosed with type 1 diabetes may have a period of remission, also called the honeymoon period or phase, where the pancreas is able to produce and secrete enough insulin to keep up with blood glucose requirements. The honeymoon period may last as long as two years.

56. A: A normal blood pressure level is <120/80 mm Hg.

57. B: Assessing the patient by using real-life scenarios immediately after the teaching session is the most effective way to ensure that the patient will be able to use these skills.

58. A: Afrezza (insulin human) may cause acute bronchospasm and should be avoided in patients with chronic lung diseases, such as chronic obstructive pulmonary disease (COPD) and asthma.

59. D: TRICARE is a health care program for military personnel, including active-duty US armed forces, National Guard or military reserve, and military family members.

60. B: Since hyperosmolar hyperglycemic syndrome (HHS) occurs in type 2 diabetes, insulin production is sufficient enough to prevent the breakdown of fat for cellular energy. Ketosis occurs only during the breakdown of fat for fuel.

61. C: Patients with hypertension and diabetes should be encouraged to do at-home blood pressure monitoring.

62. C: At least 8 hours should have passed since the last meal or drink to accurately reflect normal circulating blood levels and prevent fluctuations caused by food.

63. B: Fruits and vegetables with the skin left on are a high source of dietary fiber.

64. B: Sodium-glucose cotransporter-2 (SGLT2) inhibitors have proven benefits and are a second-line treatment of choice for reducing heart failure.

65. A: Smoothies and other liquid meal replacements are often rich in carbohydrates, leading to hyperglycemic episodes.

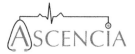

66. B: Typically, children with diabetes will be mature enough to begin managing their own diabetes regimen between the ages of 14 and 18.

67. D: If the dose for the patient is 0.15 mL, then the total number of units received is 15. 100 units/1 mL × 0.15 mL = 15 units

68. C: Employers are allowed to require a medical assessment to determine if the patient's care management may impede job performance, productivity, or safety.

69. A: Invokana (canagliflozin) is a sodium-glucose cotransporter-2 (SGLT2) inhibitor. It increases the amount of glucose excreted in the urine, putting the patient at higher risk for developing yeast infections.

70. A: Obesity is one of the primary factors in developing sleep apnea.

71. D: Waiting until after a meal to administer insulin to small children allows for flexible dosage that meets the needs of the child. This avoids having to guess how much the child will eat, which could risk causing hypoglycemia.

72. A: Elevated levels of lipids in the blood increase the risk of atherosclerosis and associated cardiovascular conditions. Patients with diabetes should have a lipid panel done immediately after diagnosis.

73. A: An A1C of 10% indicates that the patient's diabetes is not well controlled. As the patient previously responded to metformin and does not have any noted factors that could be contributing to the hyperglycemia, an increase in the dosage would likely be tried first.

74. B: Option B is the best answer choice and represents one of many goals set forth by the National DPP. Option A would be inaccurate; the CDC has set standards for a curriculum specific to a lifestyle-changing program for people who are at risk of diabetes and not for a diabetes care and education specialist (DCES). Option C is incorrect since the program is tailored towards improving the health outcomes of people who are at risk of developing type II diabetes. Option D is incorrect since the goal of the National DPP is to ensure quality diabetes prevention programs; like option C, the program is focused on people who are at risk of developing type II diabetes.

75. C: A fasting goal for patients with gestational diabetes is <95 mg/dL; however, it is important to note that a value under 60 mg/dL indicates hypoglycemia that requires treatment.

76. D: The target level for total cholesterol is <200 mg/ dL.

77. D: Amylin is responsible for regulating glucagon release and slowing gastric emptying, which causes a feeling of satiety.

78. D: Oral decongestants, such as pseudoephedrine, raise blood glucose levels by blocking insulin secretion and peripheral uptake of glucose into the cells.

79. C: Proliferative retinopathy means that in addition to the microaneurysms seen in non-proliferative retinopathy, new, abnormal blood vessels have grown, which are fragile and may bleed.

80. A: Nuts contain very little glucose, making the glycemic value near zero. All of the other foods listed are high in carbohydrates.

81. A: The abdomen injection site provides the fastest absorption of insulin.

82. A: Fibrates are an alternative to lower LDL-cholesterol when statins are not tolerated.

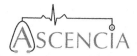

83. D: The glycemic index system is a tool that assigns numbers to foods based on that food's effect on rising blood sugar. A higher number indicates how quickly a food is digested and the glucose is absorbed, which then indicates how quickly it causes a rise in blood glucose levels.

84. A: ACE inhibitors are recommended as a first-line blood pressure treatment in patients with diabetes.

85. B: The specialist should first assess the patient's current cognitive state and ability to perform both cognitive and physical tasks. This assessment will reveal the patient's memory and abilities. Then, if appropriate, the specialist can inquire about the patient's previous management of diabetes.

86. B: Sodium-glucose cotransporter-2 (SGLT2) inhibitors have proven benefits for reducing chronic kidney disease. If kidney function is adequate, they are considered a second-line treatment of choice.

87. B: Women and persons with diabetes may not present with the typical signs of a heart attack. The signs and symptoms described may be due to a heart attack, which would need immediate, emergent care.

88. A: Early on in type 1 diabetes, a period of remission, or honeymoon phase, indicates that the child's pancreas is able to release enough endogenous insulin to manage blood glucose levels. This period typically lasts between 6 months and 2 years. In this case, the parents should anticipate that they will need to monitor and treat hyperglycemia with insulin within the next 6 months.

89. A: Lisinopril is an angiotensin-converting enzyme (ACE) inhibitor. It blocks the angiotensin-converting enzyme which prevents vasoconstriction and relaxes blood vessels.

90. D: During hyperosmolar hyperglycemic state (HHS), increased urination and hypotension can progress to intracerebral dehydration, resulting in poor cerebral blood perfusion.

91. D: During the maintenance stage, the specialist should help patients with their obstacles to meeting goals and provide guidance and encouragement.

92. D: Type 2 diabetes may require insulin as the disease progresses. An A1C of 11% would indicate uncontrolled blood sugar and the need to begin insulin.

93. D: Therapy and anti-anxiety medication are the standard recommended courses of treatment for people with anxiety.

94. C: Rhabdomyolysis is a serious medical condition which involves rapid damage to muscle tissue; it can be caused by statins.

95. A: Cortisol, an anabolic steroid, increases the rate at which glycogen breaks down and increases blood glucose levels.

96. B: Varenicline is a medication that assists with smoking cessation by reducing the effects of withdrawal and preventing the systemic effects of nicotine. Mood changes are a known side effect, and the patient should be screened for any changes or new feelings of depression.

97. C: High levels of triglycerides are associated with an increased risk of cardiovascular disease. The target level for triglycerides is <150 mg/dL.

98. B: Early recognition and treatment of any wounds on feet will prevent progression to cellulitis.

99. D: Potatoes are higher in carbohydrates and easily digested, resulting in spikes in blood glucose levels. This addition would increase the glycemic index of the overall meal. The other options would slow digestion via additional fiber and fat.

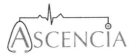

100. A: Dipeptidyl peptidase-4 (DPP-4) inhibitors suppress glucagon secretion, slow gastric emptying, and reduce overall food intake by regulating appetite.

101. D: Diabulimia, also known as eating disorder diabetes mellitus type 1 (ED-DMT1), is a type of eating disorder that involves insulin restriction in order to control weight. It is not recognized as a diagnosis in the *Diagnostic and Statistical Manual of Mental Disorders (DSM)*; however, it is sometimes classified as a purging behavior.

102. D: Because there was no harm to the patient, this scenario is considered a near-miss. It is important to always use a patient's full name and birth date for verification purposes.

103. D: An adult patient with type 2 diabetes and an A1C of 10.2% is a candidate for long-acting basal insulin or bedtime neutral protamine Hagedorn (NPH) insulin. Insulin glargine is a long-acting basal insulin and is appropriately dosed once daily in the evening.

104. B: Type 1 diabetes is characterized by three stages. In the first stage, the presence of autoantibodies in blood will reflect pancreatic damage, but the patient will be normoglycemic and not show any signs or symptoms of diabetes.

105. D: Academic assistance is not a part of the 504 plan. A 504 plan is implemented to ensure access to free public education for all students and ensures that the child's diabetes needs are met while within the public education system.

106. B: Systems-level mechanisms have been developed to identify social determinants of health (SDOH), which could help determine which factors impact treatment. Some factors that have been identified that are associated with SDOH include food insecurity, limited English proficiency, limited health literacy, low literacy, and homelessness. Social capital and community support are other factors that are associated with poorer health outcomes.

107. B: Insulin is often referred to as the "key" that allows glucose to enter cells.

108. D: Hyperthyroid exacerbations will present similarly to hypoglycemic episodes. Patients with hyperthyroidism should always check their blood sugar first prior to treating suspected hypoglycemia.

109. A: Symlin (pramlintide acetate) is an injectable antidiabetic agent. It is administered subcutaneously (sub-q) immediately prior to meals.

110. B: Most patients with type 2 diabetes do not need to follow a very low carbohydrate dietary pattern; proper carbohydrate intake helps achieve glucose regulation and glycemic control.

111. D: Pediatric patients will require frequent dose changes to adjust to increased growth and hormonal changes during puberty. Insulin requirements may also be higher than expected. Basal insulin provides a base level and will comprise approximately 50 – 60% of the total daily insulin dose, with extra coverage of bolus insulin given intermittently during the day.

112. D: Creatinine is filtered by the kidneys. A serum creatinine level over 1.2 mg/dL indicates damage to the kidneys.

113. C: The nutritionist should recognize that this age range, especially in females, is prone to developing eating disorders, including restricting food and decreasing insulin doses to avoid gaining weight.

114. A: Norvasc (amlodipine besylate) is a calcium channel blocker. It works by blocking the movement of calcium in vascular muscles, relaxing blood vessels.

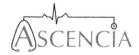

115. A: The American Diabetes Association (ADA) recommends that patients with prediabetes be screened annually for diabetes.

116. B: When dietary pattern measures are not successful, patients should be managed with the least complicated medication regimen. Since a sulfonylurea may increase the risk for hypoglycemic events, a single dose of long-acting basal insulin may be most effective in controlling this patient's blood glucose levels.

117. C: An insulin correction factor is the amount a unit of rapid-acting insulin will lower a patient's blood glucose level. One unit of rapid-acting insulin will lower this patient's BG by 30 mg/dL.

118. C: The 15-15 rule for the treatment of hypoglycemic signs and symptoms indicates the person should consume 15 grams of carbohydrates to raise blood glucose (BG) and then check BG levels after 15 minutes.

119. C: Recurrent hypoglycemic episodes can disrupt the release of epinephrine to counter hypoglycemia, which reduces common hypoglycemic symptoms, such as anxiety and tremors.

120. C: Though target ranges are adapted individually, for patients with low risk of cardiovascular disease the recommended blood pressure (BP) target is <140/90 mmHg.

121. A: Anorexia nervosa is characterized by an intense fear of gaining weight, distorted body image, and extreme calorie restriction.

122. C: Glycogenolysis occurs in the liver and is the breakdown of glycogen into glucose. Damage to the liver may disrupt this process, resulting in hypoglycemia.

123. A: A blood glucose >250 mg/dL, fruity breath, and dehydration are signs of diabetic ketoacidosis (DKA), especially in a patient with known type 1 diabetes. DKA is differentiated from other diabetes complications by the presence of ketones in the blood or urine.

124. B: The increase in blood glucose (BG) that occurs after eating stimulates the pancreas to release insulin in a biphasic release pattern with two waves.

125. C: Due to the possibility that this person may not notice injuries, especially to the feet, a thorough skin assessment should be completed to ensure that the patient's skin is intact.

126. A: An immediate outcome goal is one which can be measured immediately after instruction; these goals often demonstrate understanding of new knowledge and skills. The other options describe intermediate or post-intermediate outcomes.

127. B: Novolin R (insulin human) is a short-acting, regular insulin that reaches its peak, or maximum effect, around 3 hours after injection.

128. B: Four ounces of juice or regular soda will provide the 15 grams of carbohydrates required to sufficiently raise blood glucose and correct hypoglycemia.

129. A: Bariatric surgery can disrupt the body's ability to absorb vitamins and minerals. Iron deficiency may occur and would result in a patient feeling tired and weak. The specialist should ask if the patient has been taking supplements to ensure that vitamin and mineral needs are being met.

130. D: Trulicity (dulaglutide) is a once-weekly injectable prescription that is used to improve blood glucose levels in patients with type 2 diabetes.

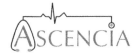

131. B: In type 1 diabetes, pancreatic beta cells produce little to no insulin, which prohibits the transport of glucose into the cells and results in a lack of energy production. The body begins to break down muscle and fat, leading to the feeling of excessive hunger, weight loss, and lethargy.

132. D: The risk for hypoglycemia rises with the complexity of the patient. With older adults, hypoglycemia is a dangerous adverse event that can increase the risk for falls, confusion, and progressive cognitive decline. To reduce the risk of inducing a hypoglycemic event, a patient with comorbidities or early-to-moderate cognitive disease should have a looser A1C target of <8% than a healthy older adult.

133. C: Oxymetazoline is delivered via nasal spray. It has less systemic exposure and is less likely to affect glucose levels.

134. C: Stocking-glove distribution is a classic sign of diabetic peripheral neuropathy (DPN). Sensory loss follows an expected pattern starting from feet, extending upward towards calves, then progressing to the hands.

135. C: The American Diabetes Association (ADA) does not recommend screening for obstructive sleep apnea in pediatric patients with type 1 diabetes.

136. B: Lifestyle modifications along with two medications are initiated for treatment when a patient's blood pressure levels are ≥160/90 mmHg.

137. A: Executive function is the ability to do everyday tasks that require planning and sequencing.

138. B: Primary interventions provide awareness, education, and screening with the goal of preventing the development of a disease. A community fair that screens people who have not been diagnosed with diabetes meets this goal.

139. D: A 65-year-old patient with diabetes and atherosclerosis is considered high risk and a candidate for high-intensity statin therapy, such as atorvastatin 40 mg.

140. B: In monogenic diabetes, glucose levels are elevated; however, there is an absence of pancreatic autoantibodies. A blood or saliva sample will be tested for the presence of defects in genes responsible for beta-cell dysfunction.

141. A: Since angiotensin-converting enzyme (ACE) inhibitors are teratogenous, they should not be used during pregnancy.

142. A: Carbohydrates in the form of sugar are inactive ingredients found in over-the-counter medications and supplements. To reduce the risk of hyperglycemia, sugar-free options should be selected.

143. B: A restrictive dietary pattern may put the patient at risk for too little protein if not monitored carefully. The goal should be to limit protein intake to 0.8 – 1.2 g/ kg/day.

144. B: The most common side effects of metformin occur in the gastrointestinal system and include nausea, vomiting, and diarrhea.

145. C: Omega-3 fatty acids are a type of polyunsaturated fatty acid that can be found in certain seeds, such as flax and chia, and in fatty fish, such as salmon and sardines.

146. D: Amylin is released along with insulin after eating. It stops the release of glucagon and slows gastric motility to elicit the feeling of being full.

Answer Key

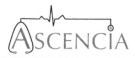

147. A: An A1C level below 7% is the target goal for most patients with diabetes and indicates good glycemic control.

148. D: The psychomotor domain encompasses motor skills. Priming the insulin pen and injecting the insulin is a complex skill that requires the patient to learn new movement patterns.

149. D: Insulin may be required in patients with type 2 diabetes with an A1C >10%, blood glucose ≥300 mg/dL, or symptoms of hyperglycemia.

150. B: Frequently seen in conjunction with type 2 diabetes, xerostomia is a condition where a lack of saliva production causes the person to experience dry mouth. Use of a xylitol-containing mouthwash or sugar-free hard candy can help alleviate dry mouth symptoms without increasing the risk of periodontal disease.

151. D: One cup of milk and half a banana each provide 15 grams of carbohydrates. This snack provides a total of 45 grams [15 + (2)15 = 45].

152. B: Glyburide is an insulin secretagogue. It works by stimulating the pancreas to make and release insulin.

153. B: Family history is the risk factor most associated with the development of diabetes.

154. A: During the third trimester, patients with diabetes may be at risk for developing diabetic ketoacidosis (DKA) at lower glucose levels. This serious complication occurs when insufficient insulin production prevents glucose use by the body's cells. It turns to the breakdown of fat as fuel, leading to the release of ketones.

155. D: The patient should inject her pen at a 90-degree angle using the dominant hand, with her fingers wrapped around the pen and the thumb free to press the knob.

156. B: The patient is showing signs of diabetes distress that are leading to barriers with self-management. Psychosocial problems among people with diabetes are very common, yet psychosocial care is an underused intervention. This intervention can identify behavioral factors, such as depression or anxiety, which may be affecting self-care and diabetes management.

157. B: The patient should be instructed to change the infusion set and infusion site every 2 – 3 days.

158. C: Dumping syndrome is a common condition in patients who have had bariatric surgery. It is exacerbated by eating meals with a high carbohydrate content that results in too much insulin being released. Postprandial hypoglycemia and rapid gastric emptying shortly after eating are hallmark signs of this condition.

159. D: An insulin vial and syringe is the most frequently used method for delivery. It is less expensive than the pen, pod, or pump and can accommodate insulin mixing.

160. B: Social workers can help patients get access to low-cost health care resources. They are also trained to help patients deal with interpersonal conflict and family dynamics.

161. B: Hyperglycemia may cause frequent and urgent urination, which may be a sign that the child requires more insulin at night. Blood sugars should be taken before bed and treated, per health care provider recommendations.

162. B: Propylthiouracil is an antithyroid agent that slows the overproduction of thyroid hormones. This medication is used to treat hyperthyroidism.

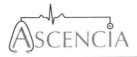

163. A: Basal insulin has a slow onset and longer duration of action. It is used to control blood glucose levels between meals.

164. D: Since the patient is requesting practice, demonstration or modeling is an effective way to teach and help the patient improve psychomotor skills. Lectures and group discussion would not meet this patient's needs.

165. A: Anhidrosis is the inability to produce adequate sweat, which can cause poor thermoregulation and compromised skin. This condition typically appears in a stocking/glove pattern.

166. C: The Association of Diabetes Care and Education Specialists (ADCES) guidelines indicate that the first follow-up should occur between two and four weeks after the patient has completed the initial session of a diabetes self-management education and support (DSMES) program.

167. B: Insulin-to-carb ratio is the amount of carbohydrates covered by one unit of rapid-acting insulin. One unit of rapid-acting insulin will cover approximately 12 – 15 grams of carbohydrates.

168. D: Dysregulation of the cardiovascular system causes symptoms such as tachycardia, hypotension, and palpitations that can affect the ability to exercise.

169. B: Coenzyme Q10 (also known as CoQ10) can lessen neuropathic symptoms in patients with diabetic

neuropathy.

170. D: This is an opportunity for the specialist to explore continued goals for the patient. An A1C of 6.4% is still elevated from normal. The patient should be educated and encouraged to continue healthy behaviors for further improvement.

171. A: A patient with type 1 diabetes should be encouraged to exercise, but there are challenges that may take some trial and error to efficiently manage blood sugars. Eating a high-carb meal or extra snack before exercising, reducing basal insulin, and treating hypoglycemic events when they arise can help patients manage their blood sugars.

172. B: A licensed practical nurse (LPN) is allowed to administer oral medications and subcutaneous insulin—not intravenous (IV) medications. The LPN should report to the registered nurse (RN) to verify the order.

173. B: Since the patient is not currently physically conditioned for intense exercise, high intensity interval training (HIIT) would not be appropriate.

174. D: Comprehensive foot exams are recommended on an annual basis for individuals who do not have peripheral neuropathy or a history of foot problems.

175. D: Driving integrated care through the health system is a proposed solution for the fragmentation of diabetes care delivery. Integrated, or horizontal integrated diabetes care, means integrating or combining primary, community, specialist, and tertiary care through similar services. Vertically integrated diabetes care is another way of delivering services or care levels by connecting with organizations. The main goal of driving integration is to have community partnerships that take responsibility for health outcomes in people with diabetes. DCESs can work with care teams and combine into their practice clinical and behavioral components to all levels of diabetes care in order to improve health outcomes.

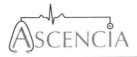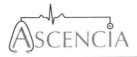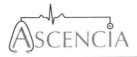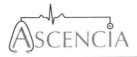

ONLINE RESOURCES

Trivium includes online resources with the purchase of this study guide to help you fully prepare for the exam.

Review Questions

Need more practice? Our review questions use a variety of formats to help you memorize key terms and concepts.

Flash Cards

Trivium's flash cards allow you to review important terms easily on your computer or smartphone.

Cheat Sheets

Review the core skills you need to master the exam with easy-to-read Cheat Sheets.

From Stress to Success

Watch "From Stress to Success," a brief but insightful YouTube video that offers the tips, tricks, and secrets experts use to score higher on the exam.

Feedback

Let us know what you think!

Access these materials at: ascenciatestprep.com/cdces-online-resources

Dear CDCES test taker,

Great job completing this study guide. The hard work and effort you put into your test preparation will help you succeed on your upcoming CDCES exam. Thank you for letting us be a part of your education journey!

We have other study guides and products that you may find useful. Search for us on Amazon.com or let us know what you are looking for. We offer a wide variety of study guides that cover a multitude of subjects.

If you would like to share your success stories with us, or if you have a suggestion, comment, or concern, please send us an email at support@triviumtestprep.com.

Thanks again for choosing us!
Happy Testing
Ascencia Test Prep Team

Made in the USA
Columbia, SC
15 February 2025

53867802R00128